The Sexual Mind

WRITTEN BY
GIRL WITH A DIRTY MIND

Published by
AUDACIOUS PRESS
http://www.audaciouspress.co.uk

The Sexual Mind
© Girl With A Dirty Mind 2011
http://www.girlwithadirtymind.com

Cover by Cathy Helms
http://www.cathyspage.com
http://www.avalongraphics.org/

Interior Photography by David Kemp
http://www.davidkphoto.com/

Interior Photographs Edited by Paul Edwards

ISBN 978-0-9563501-1-4

WITH THANKS

Thank you to everyone who believed in me through my transition from administration into writing. I give thanks to my wonderful, generous mother, Christine, special and ever supportive sister, Susie, and everyone else who supported my dream! Thank you for the blessings and guidance. You have never given up on me!

This writing path has been long and arduous, struggle after struggle financially, but I feel blessed to have a motivating mind that pushes me to continue!

To the loving Angels who filled me with faith to carry on when finances were low. Thanks for all those feathers of hope and number synchronicity that entered my life path, helping me to manifest my dreams. I know there is a divine power within us all.

To my Higher Self who has helped me follow my heart, forget about fear, and take a leap of faith to continue with this journey. Instinct is our guided sixth sense, there to serve us and keep us on the path to happiness.

The Sexual Mind is dedicated to the hidden side buried within us all.

CONTENTS

PREFACE

After thirteen years of soul searching for my ideal career, I found it in the place we, unfortunately, often look last—in myself. My prose of this easy to read guidebook flows easily from my life experiences as a masseuse, physical trainer, lover, sexual experimenter, and satisfier of my own desires.

I enjoy writing erotica from experience, and I have been lucky throughout my life to experience strong chemistry with likeminded partners. Although I found it tough to find a perfect mate for my high sex drive, I gave up and embraced my sexuality. I knew, in time, the right man would step into my life and sweep me off my feet.

I am also the type of girl who never listens to what other people say. I like to try things out for myself. A bad break up soon brought me out of my shell, and my sexual experimentation phase began.

At first, I wrote stories about my sexual adventures. It gave me confidence. I then realized my mind fitted erotica, and although not everyone can handle a confident, sexual girl like me, most of my ex-lovers liked my open sexuality. I learned then that my talents existed primarily to turn others on.

This guide is fun, motivating, and written from my perspective. I want you and your partner to reach the depths of pleasure I gained writing it. Fantastic sex is freely available to us all. Life is short, but orgasms are infinite. Effortlessly control those pleasurable endorphins at any time of the day, not only in the morning, evening, or at weekends, but during spontaneous encounters, or when the desire arises.

Why not get naughty at work? Orgasms relieve stress instantly through the release of pain reducing endorphins, and great sex will bring you closer together with your partner. Take off that shy mask, because now is the time to embrace your sexuality.

I am a very open and honest person, and I wish to share my tips and favorite foreplay methods with others. Great sex with a special partner enlivens every pore in your body and creates a memorable experience. With the right person, sex becomes magical. Put together two similar minded people with equal chemistry, and out pops explosive sex.

My break up from Jason in 2003 brought me out of my docile state. I began to experience sex as fun and pleasurable. Before Jason, sex meant nothing to me, nor did, blowjobs or masturbation. All that changed, however, after experiencing countless one-night stands. I realized sex, obviously with a chemically compatible partner, stimulated my sexuality and unleashed a wild uninhibited side I never knew existed. I continued with my experimental journey and learned sex was exciting—nothing like the habitual lovemaking I shared with Jason.

I have been single for over eight years. I do not crave sex because I have all the tools necessary to pleasure my body in numerous ways. Over the years, I have been lucky to meet a selection of great lovers who took me to the realms of desire I craved subconsciously, and I too displayed a love of unselfish sex by becoming an enthusiastic, experimental lover.

The techniques and thoughts in this guide are from experience, and I want to share my inspiring views of sex with you. Make the choice to embrace your sexual mind today.

Girl with a Dirty Mind,
February 2011

INTRODUCTION AND "RULES"

INTRODUCTION

Whether you are a sexual novice or someone who loves to experiment, you will find this guide liberating, mind opening, and certain to increase the satisfaction of you and your partner's lovemaking.

This inventive guide taps into the power of the mind to create and intensify every sexual experience. Using the mind in full force allows you to fall into sexual stimulation. The power of the mind, especially for women, makes the power of physical stimulation seem tiny. Yet pure physical stimulation is what most people base their sex lives upon.

Add mental surrender to the sexual experience, and the additional desire and need to build emotion and depth, and the urge can transcend into a sweeping tornado. Finally, the result is the increase in how ardent, extreme, eager, forceful, and satisfying your orgasms and experiences will become, building a bond between you and your partner.

Perhaps you saw a common thread in the last paragraph between the mind and mental stimulation. Your goal lies in harnessing its stimulating power and relating that power to pure physical stimulation techniques.

Yes, there are numerous physical techniques throughout this book, but they are designed in such a way to engage all the senses, lower inhibitions, raise your confidence, and open the door to your powerful mind.

Those of you willing to use the suggestions and techniques in this guide will find that you can unlock your inner self to become more experimental, in control, and free to feel and express the joys of lovemaking. By releasing your own sexual energy, you will compound your partner's level of arousal and, in turn, this will transfer back to you in a magnifying cycle of profound sexual enlightenment.

A mental sexual partnership and mutually compounding arousal is the key to reaching the heightened states of intense orgasm. It is probable that no one handed you a guide to sex when you reached puberty. So now, here it is.

With a complete lack of instruction on how to operate our highly complex sexual machines, many people are taught about guilt, insecurities, inhibitions, misinformation, and moralizing that counters our bodies' natural response to sexual stimulus.

The Sexual Mind engages all of the senses to enhance every sexual experience. Mental "baggage," however, works to demean or limit the sexual experience. An uninhibited mind makes sex more intense and enjoyable. An inhibited mind will gain the most from this guide and find the techniques liberating, taking you to an entirely new space of experience when the body combines with the mind.

The chapter on "The Power of The Mind" provides you with the necessary tools in order to free yourself from mental "baggage," increase confidence, and set you on a liberated course to reach intense orgasms.

The section on dos and don'ts will help you avoid the common turn offs that may affect you and your partner's sexuality, while at the same time, the encouraging techniques will help you and your partner enter a realm where his/her satisfaction feeds back to you. In building a self-feeding cycle, you will soar to heightened states of sexuality and beyond.

The creative sections of this guide addressing unique and advanced techniques will help to take your lovemaking out of the ordinary right from the start. The result stirs your partner out of the day-to-day routine, and lets his/her creativity add to yours.

This creates a spontaneous experience for you both, carrying you and your partner to places previously unknown. Sex is a team sport—best results release from working together.

These new discoveries invoke the power of your sexual mind to bring forth spontaneous, creative, and intense lovemaking. If you want that animal attraction—"Grrr, I want you now!—type of sex, all the tools are here. The next step to greater sexual satisfaction lies in your hands.

EMPOWER YOUR SEXUALITY

There are fun ways to empower your sexuality. The key is to expand your mind to think differently, and this is best prepared with new techniques like the "rules" detailed below.

- Experiment
- Adjust To Your Partner
- Move
- Display Self-Confidence
- Talk Filthy Or Give Your Partner Clues
- Surrender
- Reverse The Roles
- Dominate
- Play Games
- Use Sexual Aids
- Seduce Multiple Erogenous Zones
- Return The Favor
- Use The Power Of The Mind
- Do Not Limit Your Positions

Experiment: Being aware of your current sexuality drives hope to recreate a dynamic sex life. By discussing the subjects of experimentation and probing hot topics like oral sex, rubbing techniques, vibrant cybersex, stimulating phone sex, domination, and additional saucy scenes, I hope this excites you to enter a sexual phase that is equipped for discovery. Are you excited? Read more!

Adjust To Your Partner: This "rule" applies to single persons who enjoy hopping into a variety of sexual relationships. If you are timid, but your partner confident, it is still possible to create electrifying sex—by adapting to your partner's style. Follow this approach to develop confidence in your bedroom skills, which also add a tempting delight for your partner to experience. If you discover your partner's favorite fantasy that an ex-partner failed to discover, you will satisfy his/her genitals to a phenomenal degree, which then builds a sizzling memory for him/her to recall.

If you prefer not to perform oral sex, but your partner enjoys this stage of intimate foreplay, try to view it from his/her angle. From my experience, pleasing a man orally feels like one of the hottest achievements in life. To hear the steady moans slipping off his tongue, while he gasps for air waiting patiently for the next move not only enhances appreciation in him for your self-less pleasure, but creates exhilaration in your genitals too.

Move: Am I right to say that many individuals prefer enthusiasm to laziness in the bedroom? If you enjoy the action of girl-on-top, be proud and display confidence in your body language. Run your fingers over your nipples during lovemaking to titillate your partner. Alternatively, move your ass during sex to turn sweaty and frantic. An energetic sex session boosts the immune system setting off an abundance of arousing pheromones to force your partner to crave every inch of your sexy body.

If he makes love to you in missionary, add some effort by pushing your hips forward to work the ass. Make every effort to step out of your comfort zone to surprise him. Show him you are the total opposite of ordinary. Men are visual creatures, so if you choose to masturbate, it is quite possible that he WILL grow aroused.

Here are a couple of tips for men. Women crave touch; kiss her lips, nibble her ears, plant flirty butterfly kisses on her neck, breasts, and between her sticky thighs. Another great benefit I should mention is the fact that s/he will view you in a different light, which will enhance any sex life. Displaying a new side of your sexuality, preferably when you feel kinky, may prove to be a major role in the transformation of your sex life.

Display Self-Confidence: Confidence is paramount in order to build a satisfying sex life. If you have the available freedom and optimism, a great time to make love is during the day. Do not worry about the natural sunlight hitting your flaws; these areas do not turn off your partner sexually. Men are grateful to view a naked curvy figure, so inhale a cleansing breath and exhale any negativity you feel inward.

Quietly declare positive statements to retrain your mind to think positively. Any type of negativity toward yourself—procrastination, anger, hate, impatience, lack, and blame is detrimental to your sexual confidence. Remind yourself that attraction comes naturally, and he loves you unconditionally. Men love a confident woman who is proud of her figure and displays an enthusiastic side during sex.

Masturbation, continuous moans of feedback, and filthy talk favors highly. Does this sound like useful information, yet you still suffer with self-confidence issues? Take each day as a positive step and do not disclose this information to friends. If every woman had a stick thin supermodel figure, life would lose its natural zest, would you agree?

The majority of men love a curvy figure to grab onto. If you are blessed with a curvy ass and hourglass hips, count yourself lucky. Any figure looks fabulous dressed in colorful fashion, and confidence is the key to sexiness. Embrace a little fat on the bones! Fat is necessary to warm the body and cushion the internal organs. If you ever do alter the shape of your body through diet or exercise, do it only for yourself—never another.

In the past, I received a nasty jibe about my healthy size twelve figure. Although I experienced great kinky sex with the six-foot eccentric Virgo, his judgment about my not-as-toned-as-a-supermodel thighs super-inflated his ego, but hurt my feelings. Believe me girls, I am sure you are with me when I state that any jibe about looks or dress size is forever stored in the subconscious mind and ready to manifest whenever your ego requires a little playful fun. His sudden comment highlighted the arrogant side that he failed to spot in himself. I left him in a state of disbelief after dominating him, blindfolding him, and giving him one of the best blowjobs of his life. Creating a reminiscent experience is always the best way to create fireworks in an ex-lover's mind. A year later, he wrote an explicit short tale to try to entice me over to Egypt (where he works as a diver). Sadly, it failed to work its magic!

A deep penetrative position e.g. doggy style provides you with the opportunity to display your curvy ass—perfect if your partner is a butt man. Show him how much you enjoy his lovemaking with enthusiastic moans. Do you prefer it harder? If so, dominate his mind with explicit words.

What do men view as positive and sexy in the bedroom, you may wonder—enthusiasm, role-play, domination, deep satisfying moans, masturbation, confidence, and a love of self-less pleasure? These skills are highly favorable.

Talk Filthy or Give Your Partner Clues: A self-less partner expresses how s/he loves to be rubbed, the depth of penetration required, and the sharing of his/her favorite foreplay techniques. Tell or show your partner what turns you on. Is a loud groan considerable enough feedback for your partner, or does s/he require additional dirty phrases to learn more about your needs?

I am confident that your partner will love this "rule" even if only to discover the inner workings of the female mind. What men crave more than ever is to pleasure a partner with a real orgasm. Therefore, feedback is necessary to help him become a satisfying lover. Without feedback, a man will exert effort to supply your body with ample pleasure, but with enthusiastic feedback his confidence will rise to an incredible level.

A real orgasm feels nothing like a fake one. Do you want to fake another orgasm after experiencing the warm waves of endorphins brushing through your body and mind during a real climax? Do not give him another excuse to fake your pleasure. For most women, the time it takes to orgasm averages twenty minutes. The body enters a tense period where the need to rush and release is a primal reason why most women still fake orgasm. If you fake an orgasm, yet he achieves climax, this could leave you feeling very unsatisfied sexually. However, you have full liberty over your sex life, and you can change the rules at any point.

Men must remain aware that the majority of women require encouragement, relaxation, and adequate time. With appropriate foreplay, arousal will stimulate each nerve ending perfectly. Throughout this guide, the various tips and techniques should motivate you to experience solo-pleasure, give you more than enough confidence to masturbate in front of your partner, and guide you into self-less oral loving.

How can you embrace your sexuality if you have never before stimulated your genitals singly? Starting today, begin a journey with your sexuality through masturbation...and practice regularly. If you prefer not to use your fingers, use a satisfying toy to stimulate your genitals. Once you allow guilt to subside, performing solo sex for the first time creates a newfound liberation.

Do not rush your orgasmic pleasure—take your time. Carefully brush your fingers over your body and discover the fantasy or fetish, which excites your genitals. Use your sexual mind to create depth in your fantasy, and then rub yourself with alternate paced strokes.

If you feel confident after orgasm, tell or show your partner how you love to be touched—I guarantee his penis will rise if you follow this tip. If this "rule" feels new to you, take it slowly. Not everyone is a fan of explicit talk, but sexual experience will develop only if you and your partner are willing to put in the time and necessary effort to build those fireworks. Foreplay can enter new realms of experimentation, but it is better to keep the secret between just you and your partner. If you feel a new sense of fervency after the exchange of filthy chat, feel proud and smile inward, but do not disclose your newfound sexuality to the local gossip. There are certain people who revel in creating tension between happy couples. This may be through a negative expression of jealousy or judgment, but it is certainly not through love.

Sex does not always have to take place in the bedroom—it can begin anywhere. Experiment in the bathroom or kitchen, but keep the liaison secret. The time you spend with a partner is yours to cherish, so turn those special occasions into fond memories.

Surrender: Forget about your partner's pleasure and surrender to the pleasure that is on offer to you. If you love to perform oral sex on each other, make a choice to give in to his/her charms and do not fight for control or feel selfish about the scene. This is not weak; it is a declaration that you enjoy your partner's dominance.

Taking control of a partner is hot! If you only have an interest in vanilla sex, but your partner has kinky expressions of interest, do not dismiss this vision. Become the self-less lover s/he craves. Discuss the scene in depth with a partner and experiment with new concepts to alter your sex life. Do these ideas excite the genitals? If so, embrace your body and offer it as a pleasurable tool for your partner to worship for a set period. Swap roles and offer the same pleasure. Continue with the surrendering role-play regularly to light up your inner spark of curiosity, altering the way you view sex forever.

Reverse The Roles: Who is the usual initiator of sex in your relationship? Are you shy and scared of embracing your sexuality, thus forcing your partner to consistently make the first move? Alternatively, do you want to change, yet require additional self-confidence? This "rule" is challenging but also a beneficial way to create a profound change in how you view your current sexuality. Reverse the roles without feeling a sense of fear or desperation.

Plan the day in detail, if it helps to reduce your overall anxieties, e.g. surprise him when he arrives home from work by pinning him against the wall and seducing him with explicit words and touch, or cover your figure in sexy lingerie to make his eyes pop out of his head on entry.

A straightforward way to distract his attention onto you would be to excite him with explicit calls or texts during the day. You do not have to masturbate to create his excitement, but sound convincing. Experimenting with naughty thoughts during the day is liberating and sure to invoke the sexual side hidden within your partner, which may only pop out at night when you spend time alone together.

Most men have many sexual thoughts on a daily basis, but work and business issues can easily distract his attention. Caress your nipples and send him a naughty picture. It is easy to excite a man with choice words, but it's even more exciting to play out the fantasy for real when he walks through the door.

Dominate: Take control of your partner's sexuality through domination. This "rule" is daring and hot, and a woman taking control of a man is a common fantasy that most men would love to experience in reality. There are countless ways to awaken a partner's rampant side. One example is to tie his wrists together, blindfold him, and use an array of materials to stimulate his skin. If you feel extra daring, use toys.

Douse your body in natural pheromones (see the chapter on "Attraction and Scents"), and dab your scent on the hot spots he loves—nape of the neck, behind the ears, backs of the knees, and between the breasts. Dress in sexy lingerie or a rubber/latex suit to draw his senses into the mood of domination. This form of role-play will draw out your experimental side, plus you will look every inch the perfect playmate through his eyes.

Play Games: Experiment with your body and learn to love masturbation. Solo masturbation is horny, sensuous, and expands your self-awareness of arousal. Do you prefer to circle your clitoris with one or two fingers, or run a couple of fingers up and down or side-to-side frantically? The penis can be stroked in various ways. Remember to breathe during masturbation. Holding the breath creates anxiety and tension, and can prolong an orgasmic release.

The practice of inhaling and exhaling deep breaths during foreplay and masturbation is productive, and builds intense orgasms that are far stronger than the norm. Do you like to rub your clitoris or penis to the edge of orgasm and control the pleasure so you are able to create a stronger release? When your body enters this highly orgasmic realm, your sexuality will rise to rampant, building amazing satisfaction.

Use Sexual Aids: Gather your sexual tools ready to use on a partner. Blindfolds, handcuffs, chains, vibrators, anal toys, lubrication, sexy outfits, food, and silk scarves are all fun tools that will cause diverse pleasures in everyone. Foreplay can be as imaginative or as sexy as you choose it to be.

A slippery sensation on the body during foreplay can feel incredibly erotic. It may mess up the sheets, but when the sexual mind heightens in arousal it generates a strong sensation in the genital area. Strawberries and cream are the perfect combination to use during food play. Edible massage oils and ice cream also create multiple sensations on the skin.

If you decide to experiment with sexual aids to heighten your sex life, but you have never before displayed a kinky side, this "rule" exhibits mystery to arouse your partner on several levels. Sexual gadgets and vibrators are perfect to use during foreplay and penetration. Used on your partner, toys are helpful for couples who do not enjoy giving oral loving. Online sex shops sell fun items ranging from chocolate shaped genitals and fruity massage oils to anal beads and rabbit vibrators. The extensive collection of sex toys could astound you.

Seduce Multiple Erogenous Zones: Throughout this guide, I include an A to Z of hot spots to excite in the body, most of which include the basic areas—lips, ears, neck, and genitals. Others are less well-known erogenous zones; whereas other hot spots may make you flinch, especially when you learn that the armpit— obviously when clean—is a hot spot to stimulate on a man.

The back of the knees is another hot spot to tease in both parties. The tailbone or coccyx (lower back) is another area to stroke, which awakens the genital region. Both the skin and the mind are the two hottest erogenous zones in the body that most people overlook.

Return The Favor: Pleasuring your partner may not be the first thing that springs to mind during any sexual activity, but covering his/her face in pleasure can feel more enjoyable than receiving gratification. A true sexual bond creates excitement and pushes your mind to furnish your partner with self-less pleasure. If the desire is to become a better lover, you must first give to receive pleasure. Please read the later chapter on "Oral Sex" to find out how to drive your partner crazy.

Do you loathe oral sex? If this is your truth, ask yourself why you feel this way? Do you find the taste revolting, or do you view it as a "dirty" or "sinful" act? After a bath or shower, how can you excuse oral sex? Beside the pleasure bestowed upon your partner, there are multiple benefits to gain. For example, oral sex prevents a double chin, burns calories, and excites you to become more experimental. Did I also mention that you would look amazing through his eyes?

The longer your tongue, lips, and fingers work the penis, the more effortless it is to enter the fat burning zone to burn off excess calories.

Use The Power of Your Mind: The mind is the most potent tool of existence in the world today, plus it is the master of erogenous zones. Used wisely, the mind can heighten any sexual experience. I am confident that most of you reading this guide would love to build and achieve stronger orgasms.

Play with the five wonderful senses—scent, taste, sight, sound, and touch. Heighten the senses in your partner by inhibiting one sense for another. For example, blindfold your partner and every time you touch, kiss, or fondle the skin, his/her mind will heighten every sensation. Diminish any one of the five senses to instantaneously revive power in another. This will create hours of stirring foreplay between you both.

Do Not Limit Your Positions: Challenge your body in how it achieves orgasm. Are you happy with missionary sex, or have you not yet experienced adventurous positions? If so, step out of your comfort zone and surprise yourself.

Try not to be predictable either. Give into your partner's pleasure without feeling the worry to return the same—gratification can be offered hours later. Three to six quickies equals a marathon session; sex does not always have to be a two-hour romp. If you prefer quickies[1] next to longer lovemaking sessions, surrender to his/her moves, and enjoy the pleasure bestowed upon your genitals until you reach a powerful climax.

THE POWER
HIDDEN WITHIN

THE POWER OF THE MIND

The mind is the most powerful erogenous zone in the body. If you use it to focus on your sexuality and mood, it will heighten every experience. Do you want to achieve supercharged intense orgasms? The key is to tap into the extraordinary power of the mind.

Unbelievably, the average person has forty thousand thoughts per day. How many of those thoughts are positive, negative, or sexually related? Think about the various decisions you make throughout the day. Instead of focusing on fear or guilt, use your mind to seek solutions. With its infinite power, the mind holds the solution to all your problems.

How do you view your life at this very minute? Can you state ten positive phrases to describe your life? However long it takes to discover the ten illuminating statements, experiment with this exercise and continue to focus on the same phrases until they melt into the subconscious. It feels amazing to journey through life experiencing new emotions and thrills, but your current reality is created through your past thoughts.

Remember of the power contained within the human mind and be aware of every thought, whether positive or negative. If it is the latter, turn it around in a second with a positive affirmation e.g. I choose to focus on positive thoughts now. Even more powerful would be to ask a motivating question, i.e. How can I help my mind to think more positively now.

If your sex life is monotonous, you can alter it by changing your thought pattern. The mind makes it easy. Arousal can hit a man after only seconds of watching a pornographic movie or reading an explicit story. The mind absorbs all sensual images and explicit words as if by magic.

Some thoughts manifest immediately, whereas others require patience and trust. If you are precise about your sexual thoughts and fantasies, and have a horny partner to match those experiences, use your supercharged mind to your advantage.

Think about how horny you will feel when your mind is re-focused to think sexually most of the time? Think of all the ways in which you would arouse your partner, or fantasize of the sexual techniques that your mind and body have yet to experience? Do you feel embarrassed and shameful to think about them, or are you ready to alter your sexuality by questioning its current level.

Dismiss the negative aspects of your mind, which want you to conform to religious or non-sexual practices. Take control and unleash your sexual mind. Try to step into that realm of the unknown where anything is possible. You want to enter a state of clarity where it takes only seconds to reach arousal.

Surely there was a point in your relationship when you experienced the hottest sex of your life? How did you reach that stage and supercharge your mind? Did you image a hot fantasy starring your favorite movie hero, or visualize a thrilling threesome? Without sexual thoughts in the mind, the body cannot reach arousal.

It may sound straightforward, but not everyone is able to stimulate the sexual part of his/her mind so easily. It could stem from religious beliefs or an upbringing that described sex as a sin. If you believe in something, but you are told it is wrong, you have been "brainwashed" into guilt and restraint. I used to believe that masturbation was wrong. I thought I'd end up in hell being pricked up the ass with a pitchfork, but I questioned why I believed those concepts and changed my beliefs. Solo sex is one of life's only free pleasures; why should that be wrong? Hell is a fictional place created only in the mind through fear.

In any loving relationship, forget about what other people taught you about sex, and make up your own rules. Experiment with your partner sexually to heighten each of the five senses and build rapture.

Most individuals enjoy the communication and sharing of sexual thoughts. An arousing but detailed fantasy may be enough to cause an orgasm in a large number of women—a prime example of the mind's potency.

When the mind achieves arousal through words, thoughts, and images, the nerve endings receive stimulation, which then arouses the genitals. Test this theory by focusing all thought and feeling onto how you reach arousal without the need to get naked with a partner. Describe how you want to touch him, and then allow him to whisper his descriptive fantasy beside your ear (another hot erogenous zone). How does his description affect your body? Is your skin now super-sensitized? Do dirty words affect your genitals? Arouse each other into a mad frenzy where you can focus on nothing but hot sex with your partner.

Communication is paramount throughout all levels of a relationship. You must be able to share strong emotions of love and discuss your intimate desires with your partner, including your favorite sexual positions, and how you crave touch.

Read the chapter on "Seduction Techniques" to titillate the mind into sexual experimentation. Use sexual aids like vibrating toys and sticky ice cream to tease every nerve ending in the body. With the appropriate time focused on foreplay to create stirring pleasure, you will both reach exciting depths of ecstasy during sex.

Consider using an array of tools to pleasure your partner in exhilarating ways. I believe that giving pleasure to another is an act of unconditional love. Accept the pleasure when it is returned to you, but always try to focus on your partner's desire. Perhaps you and your partner share the same outlook. To become a good lover, you must first experiment with techniques that will fulfill his/her pleasure.

Accessing the power of the mind to boost the sex life is easy. Nor does it require a partner by your side. Hot foreplay can occur over the phone, via cybersex, or through text sex. Whatever your favorite mode of messenger, allow it to turn a fantasy into sexual suggestion or domination.

If the sharing of sexual thoughts with your partner feels strange, push through those boundaries one step at a time. Eventually, you will come face to face with your inner minx.

It is easy to boost your sexuality by focusing on foreplay, not only in the bedroom, but in every other area of your life too. I discuss the five senses throughout this guide, however there is another I like to call the "sixth sense of sexuality"——focusing the mind on the body part receiving pleasure in order to create excitement.

To reach that passionate core situated in your mind, you must first lock out all doubt, insecurity, and the rest of the world. An example of this would be to let your partner dominate you. Focus on his hands, tongue, lips, or fingers teasing your skin. How does it make you feel? Hot, sexy, and desperate to feel him inside you perhaps?

If any thoughts unrelated to sex enter your mind, be aware and erase them immediately. If additional sexy thoughts slip into your mind, concentrate on those saucy images. Continue to focus on your pleasure; think of nothing else. By relaxing with intentional thoughts on your given pleasure, you will find it easier to achieve intense orgasms.

When a sexual problem occurs, most individuals write into a newspaper or magazine for advice e.g. I feel tense because I cannot achieve a real orgasm. If you struggle to reach orgasm, do you search inward at your thoughts and discover how they could be harboring your current sex life? Stress, bodily confidence issues, and having no ability to focus on your own pleasure can make it difficult to orgasm. If you fall into this category, you may panic because of the struggle to climax and fake an orgasm instead. If you focused on your pleasure, rather than destroying insecurities, and learn to inhale deep breaths, the self-conscious issues will gradually fade.

The unconscious mind soaks up all good or bad thoughts like a sponge. If you focus on problems with worry, you can make the situation feel worse than it already is. Life is based on the choices that your mind focuses upon. It will give you exactly what you think about. If you dwell on problems rather than solutions, more problems will manifest into your life. If you do not understand what I am saying, educate yourself on the law of attraction.

Stress is a prime factor of negativity and interferes with arousal. Now is the time to give it a kick up the backside and refuse to let it alter your sexual relationship with a partner.

Appropriate time spent with a partner equals a spicy sex life. Make no excuse to get close to him/her. If your prime aim is to experience a real orgasm, you must first learn to relax by inhaling deep breaths. When the mind is relaxed and focused on its goal, it is easier to reach orgasm. Gentle hair pulling and massage is soothing for the mind.

Do not try to force an orgasm as this could manifest as tension. However, do focus on compelling desire. In my later chapter on "Hot Foreplay Methods," I discuss the importance of focusing the mind on the present moment during incredible foreplay. When your partner is caressing your body, relax and enjoy every second of the experience. Use the power of your mind to focus on the sensation to endure mind-blowing orgasms.

DOS AND DON'TS TO CREATE SEXUAL ECSTASY

- **Do** give your partner plenty of clues about how you like to be touched.
- **Do** experiment with every sexual encounter.
- **Do** learn to enjoy giving pleasure.
- **Do** experiment with exotic positions.
- **Do** indulge in the art of erotic kissing.
- **Do** tap into the power of the mind.
- **Do** experiment with domination.
- **Do** use silks and other fabrics to enhance the sensations felt during foreplay.
- **Do** use toys on yourself and your partner.
- **Do** limit the senses.
- **Do** masturbate alone and in front of your partner.
- **Do** learn to talk dirty.
- **Do** give in to the reciprocal pleasures.
- **Do** display enthusiasm and confidence in the bedroom.
- **Do** learn to admire your body.
- **Do** use the tongue to heighten your partner's pleasure during acts of foreplay.
- **Do** use the art of body language to flirt with your partner.
- **Do** explore the art of touch with your hands.
- **Do** choose sensuous locations other than the bedroom. For example, anywhere outdoors, on the patio, in a hot tub, and swaying in a hammock etc.
- **Do** focus 100% pleasure on your partner.
- **Do** surprise your partner with foreplay.
- **Do** allow your mind and body to feel every surge of pleasure from your partner before exploding with an orgasm.
- **Do** touch, rub, tickle, tease, and stroke.

- **Do** complement your partner on his/her body, his/her reactions, and his/her performance.
- **Do** experiment with toys.

- **Don't** just lie there.
- **Don't** be selfish in the bedroom. Learn to enjoy giving selfless pleasure.
- **Don't** always turn off the light during foreplay and sex.
- **Don't** cover up your body; show it off.
- **Don't** make love in just one position—become experimental with others.
- **Don't** be quiet; be vocal.
- **Don't** use your teeth during oral sex.
- **Don't** be shy about showing off your spontaneous side.
- **Don't** let stress get in the way of your sexual endeavors.
- **Don't** have quickies all the time.
- **Don't** over think every move.
- **Don't** plan a sexual encounter allow it to come naturally.
- **Don't** roll over after orgasm.

THE SEXUAL MIND QUIZ

Be as honest as you can with this simple quiz and read the results on the following pages. If you are not happy with the result, be adventurous and learn new methods that will boost your sex life.

The twelve questions are designed to pinpoint how experimental you are in your current sexual relationship. The questions are not meant to offend, but rather to intrigue you into viewing sex as an enjoyable act, which releases stress and brings you closer to your partner.

Tick the answers that correspond best to your first thought. If an answer does not spring to mind at first thought, go with your instinct, then read on for a summary of your frequent circled answers.

1.   How often do you and your partner get sexual?

Not very frequently, only on special occasions.	A
Three to five times per month.	B
We have sex more than once a week.	C
Daily—we are unable to keep our hands off each other.	D

2.   What about sexual experimentation. How often does this occur?

Sex is always in the same old missionary position.	A
Make up sex after an argument is the last time we got kinky.	B
I like to dominate my partner, but only on special occasions.	C
Regularly with porn, erotica, group sex, and sex toys.	D

3.   How do you regard foreplay?

A little kissing and vanilla lovemaking.	A
Twenty minutes of genital stroking ahead of intercourse.	B
Massage, passionate kisses, and domination.	C
Foreplay can be so erotic between us; it often feels better than sex.	D

4. **Have you ever experimented sexually out of the bedroom?**

Sex remains only in the bedroom and always with the lights off.	A
We had sex on the beach on our honeymoon night.	B
Occasionally, we make love on the sofa.	C
Yes, we make love whenever and wherever the mood strikes us.	D

5. **Do you ever masturbate?**

No because I would end up in hell.	A
Never, this is a sin against my religion.	B
I have experimented once or twice, yes.	C
I masturbate alone and with my partner regularly.	D

6. **Do you fantasize or have you ever participated in a real life fantasy with your partner?**

No, I have no idea of what to image.	A
Only in my mind and with my favorite celebrity.	B
I do fantasize, but I have not yet turned it into reality.	C
My partner and I discuss and star in fantasies on a regular basis.	D

7. **Do you like to give/receive oral sex?**

No way, that's borderline dirty.	A
I receive it yes, but I would never return the favor.	B
Only on special occasions will he get the full works.	C
All the time and its the reason why my chin remains taut.	D

8. **Are you able to read the body language of others?**

No, I have no idea of what to look for.	A
A smile and a little eye contact is the start of a friendly connection.	B
Conversation, stance, and mirroring displays attraction.	C
Yes, I am a magnet for attraction.	D

9. **Are you a good flirt?**

What is a flirt?	A
I am a bit rusty and need some tips.	B
I have worked my flirtatious magic on partners in the past.	C
Oh yes, I know how to flirt to my advantage to get what I want.	D

10. **How often do you experiment with sexual positions?**

Not really, we hardly have sex.	A
Does missionary count?	B
Occasionally I like to get on top.	C
We make love in all kinds of exotic positions.	D

11. **Where did you and your partner meet?**

Somewhere religious.	A
In a library.	B
At my local nightclub or similar venue.	C
At a theme park, racing circuit, or other spontaneous event.	D

12. **What is the hottest text message you have ever sent to your partner?**

Should we eat desserts tonight?	A
I love you, sexy.	B
I bet you can't wait to see me wearing sexy lingerie tonight.	C
You, me, and a bottle of baby oil tonight.	D

Mostly As: Your sex life is more traditional than experimental. You must learn to think out of the box. Try to rid the mind of the perception that sex is sinful or only to conceive a child? Sex is designed to be fun. Masturbation is perfectly healthy and a natural stress-reliever. Solo-sex also encourages your mind to fantasize. I hope that this guide helps to unleash all of your carnal instincts. Read each tip and technique in this guide to help you move into a new level of sexual awareness. I recommend you feed positive statements/affirmations into your subconscious. Read the chapters on "Masturbation," "Orgasms," Desire," "Body Language," and "Hot Foreplay Methods."

Mostly Bs: Perhaps you have experimented sexually with your partner in the past or looked for ways to build your sex life into something fun. However, you must incorporate more foreplay into your sex life to build intense orgasms and a deeper connection with your partner. Practice daily affirmations to rid the mind of guilt. Please refer to the later chapters on "Fun Sexual Tips," "Masturbation," "Desire," "Oral Sex," and "Hot Foreplay Methods."

Mostly Cs: You two are hot! You have experimented with most of the techniques listed throughout this guide. Educate yourself on body language and telepathic suggestion and you will be well on your way to becoming a God/Goddess. I recommend that you read the chapters on "Hot Foreplay Methods," "Oral Sex," and "Masturbation."

Mostly Ds: You two share a very spicy sex life. This guide may offer some variations on foreplay, but you two sure do love to experiment. You have built up a red-hot sex life that contains reciprocated desire, solo and mutual masturbation, self-less pleasure, oral sex, fantasies, foreplay, and erotic sexual positions. Experiment with each of the foreplay methods, and if the positions are nothing out of the ordinary, why not design a workout of your own?

THE SEXUAL MIND

This guide is designed to heighten the mind of both you and your partner by focusing on a move to cause his/her pleasure. Through feedback, an enthusiastic writhing body, moans, thrusts, and intense orgasms, you communicate sexual arousal together. This feedback instigates deeper penetrations and causes a craving that makes you want to furnish your partner with forthcoming pleasure.

Physically display any form of devotion—a faster rolling ass, an orgasm, or a loud exhilarating sigh. Whatever feedback you choose to focus on, make sure you work with the mind and body to demonstrate exactly how much you love his/her moves.

This self-feeding cycle builds passion, desire, and encourages an orgasm that is out of the ordinary—an explosion that not only causes a few dribbles or seconds of pleasure, but a deeper, fulfilling climax. With a focus on foreplay and its many techniques, this guide will teach you how to limit the senses, build patience, create supremacy and lust, while providing you with a selection of techniques to help the body experience awe-inspiring pleasure.

Choose to focus on the pleasure of your partner without expectation for the same in return. By providing this pleasure, the excitement you offer your partner will be from an unconditional state of affection. The wonderful sensations you present through foreplay, together with your partner's enthusiastic feedback should spur you on to furnish him/her with more pleasure in a self feeding frenzy.

This is sure to excite women who receive only a quick flick of the clit during foreplay. If you feel dissatisfied with your lovemaking, or you fake orgasm frequently, be bold and confess of your substandard pleasure. Mention that you would like him to focus on your body without you feeling under pressure to orgasm in five or ten minutes.

Fingertip stimulation or use of a feather or piece of silky material on the many erogenous zones will arouse the nerve endings effortlessly. If this technique does not excite you, ask your partner to stimulate other sensitive areas. If you still feel no satisfaction during or after the act, then your partner receives no reciprocal pleasure. Magnificent orgasms are worth the wait.

If your lover is unrestrained during lovemaking, ask him/her to slow down to create a unique and harmonious scene. No woman wants to experience a quickie ALL the time. However, women do crave an emotional and mental connection, which includes foreplay, kisses, caressing, licking, stroking, and the finale of a REAL orgasm.

Throughout this guide, I discuss oral sex, orgasms, sexual aids, masturbation, and I also highlight a number of hot foreplay methods that have worked well for me. There is also the "Sexual Workouts" chapter detailing the easy lovemaking positions to the more advanced. I learnt to satisfy my body through masturbation and sex, and I hope this guide helps you experience the same. Sufficient sex tones the body and creates a deep sweat, ridding the body of deathly toxins, while oral sex prevents a double chin. Finally, orgasms release natural painkillers, which help to relieve menstrual cramps, breast pain, and migraines.

For some women, it may be difficult to step out of the "virginal" image. If you want your partner to view you as a deity, you must first learn to view yourself as a powerful Goddess. You can release your virginal image and invoke your natural Goddess through solo experimentation.

Most couples marry through love and to spend their lives together until death parts them. Contrary to the belief, even a solid marriage requires hard work. Sex retains prime importance for most couples. Therefore, it is important to keep the relationship alive with communication, foreplay, trust, love, and experimentation. Spontaneity will set off the fireworks and prove that your marriage or relationship is built on intimacy and trust.

Due to work issues and other restraints, it may be difficult for a couple to find the time to experience marathon sex sessions, or spend a full romantic evening together focusing on foreplay. Within this guide is a brief summary of the male/female anatomy, the hottest erogenous zones to excite, and foreplay methods to heighten the senses.

If you answered the questions in the last chapter honestly, then you should now know your current "sexual rating." Is it poor, adequate, good, or steamy? If your answers equaled better than average, this guide will motivate you to intensify your sexuality. On the other hand, if your rating was adequate or poor, you have a lot of work to do inside yourself to alter your mindset to focus sexually. With the appropriate time, dedication, and an open mind, this guide aspires to change the way you view sex forever. It will help to clear away unresolved insecurities, while also liberating your mind.

Do you experiment with masturbation alone, or do you include your partner in the action? Have you ever wondered how it would feel to try an exhilarating sexual position to awaken the genitals? Do you ever imagine how it would feel if your partner tied you up with a silk scarf and dominated you for hours? If you answered a significant yes to one or more of the above, or you have already experimented with domination, fantastic! If not, I hope to furnish your mind with techniques on how to take your sex life from mundane to hot hot hot!

Would you agree that for most people, part of his/her twenty-four hour day is filled with stress and other obstacles usually relating to finance? Work and debt problems dominate the mind, and the motivation to get kinky with a partner then becomes ancient history. Are you still in the mood for sex when there are multiple responsibilities that can take up far too much of your time? Life should focus less on stress and more on the fun elements of building fond memories with a partner. Marital life and long-term relationships deserve effort in all areas, including intimacy and sex.

If the thought of experimenting with new techniques has never entered your mind, this guide offers an array of fun tips on how to work your partner into a frenzied state, while also unleashing those deep levels of intimacy already within you. I also include a section on masturbation to help you achieve orgasm. There is nothing weak about fulfilling your own sexual desires. I believe that fun should be the focal point of the day, rather than fatigue causing negative stress.

Slow, sensual sex is gratifying during the moment, but why not unleash that animalistic side of yourself that you have kept hidden for far too long. In the chapter on "Hot Foreplay Methods," I summarize each technique and then offer easy ways on how to heighten the senses. This may include limiting a sense to highlight another, exciting one or more of the many sensitive erogenous zones, or touching/kissing/caressing and nibbling with a generous measure of foreplay.

This guide will help both parties to open up his/her sexual mind to view foreplay as much more than simple gratification. The human mind is powerful and must be educated with focus and stimulation to heighten the senses. To build a powerful connection sexually, you must first develop a love of foreplay and add the appropriate efforts to satisfy your partner. If the aim is to build sensational intimacy with your partner, you **must** focus time and effort on foreplay. The sexual heights you will both experience are worth the efforts.

I am confident that most of you reading this guide would love to experience deeper, fulfilling orgasms. While a quickie often releases a man's ejaculation and orgasm, it can be very limiting for a woman. Are you one of the many women who choose to admit this fact?

If I told you that regular foreplay and experimentation could turn you multi-orgasmic, would you believe me? Do you feel intrigued about how to go from adequate to sizzling hot? If yes, stick with me.

SCENE 1

You and your partner are snuggling together in bed. He starts to caress your body, and you grow slowly aroused. You know that foreplay does not normally last long, so you give in and fake another orgasm. He gets his fulfilling orgasm through penetration, and you are growing sick of him always having the sexual power.

The Problem: Simple, your partner wears the trousers in the bedroom, and you give in too easily by faking an orgasm that offers you no sexual gratification. Have you forgotten about your own carnal desires? He already believes he is a sex God because of the faked orgasm in you he believed to be real. Alter the situation by stating that you NOW crave more than a mere five minutes of foreplay. Let him work for his pleasure, and do not feel guilty about how long it takes for you to reach orgasm. A fake orgasm strokes his ego, but does nothing to pleasure your body. The body involuntary shakes; the vagina contracts, endorphins flood the body, the cheeks and chest flush, and the breaths turn shallow and uncontrollable during a real climax.

Take Charge: Turn on the light, sit on top of your partner's body or face (if you feel extra confident), and masturbate. This will turn him rock hard in seconds and create a memorable sight. Do not worry about the time it takes for you to reach arousal and climax. Ask your partner to describe how he would pleasure you while you masturbate, and imagine that fantasy is real. Never confess of a faked orgasm to a man, even during an argument. This will cause a massive blow to his ego. Instead, allow him to watch you masturbate until you achieve a mind-blowing climax. If you have never before stroked your clitoris alone or in front of your partner, let him stroke you to ecstasy through masturbation and/or oral sex. Give him constant feedback on every sensation you feel inside your body. When s/he hears your real moans of joy, you will feel mutual excitement about spending time together and experience REAL orgasms.

How It Improves Your Sex Life: Displaying confidence is sexy. Most men would love to watch a girl masturbate. Pleasuring your body and allowing your partner to watch first teaches him the exact tricks that "get you off." Your partner will then aspire to make you cum wilder. During foreplay and oral loving, every man has the secret hope that his partner's orgasm is REAL In fact, faking orgasm teaches a man nothing.

SCENE 2

You have just given her a hot orgasm orally, but she is not a big fan of fellatio.[2] Obviously, you crave oral sex in return, yet you are afraid to request the same in case it causes a rift with her. You make love to your partner and climax through penetration.

The Problem: Your partner cannot read your mind and know of your desire for oral loving. Your sex life is beginning to feel routine and drab. In some areas, you crave fun elsewhere, yet you love your partner far too much to act unfaithful. You have tried to discuss the situation with her, but she ignores your plea, which makes you feel even more desperate and unfulfilled.

Take Charge: You must explain to her of your need to feel some sexual gratification orally after giving her that exact same pleasure. If she loves your lips and tongue sucking on her clitoris, yet she will not perform the same act in return, it may be time to offer an ultimatum. Refuse to perform oral sex again unless she gives you an enthusiastic blowjob in return. If you strike it lucky and she gives in to your desire, this is your opportunity to show and tell your partner how you like to masturbate. If she feels intimidated by your sexually forward vibe, reassure her that you would love any exciting efforts. Is she worried about swallowing sperm perhaps? If so, keep a box of tissues close to the bedside and hand her one when you feel ready to burst. In addition, state that fellatio burns over five hundred calories per thirty minutes, and she will love to get kinky on your manhood.

How It Improves Your Sex Life: It is perfectly okay to have an opinion about sex and request self-less pleasure from your partner. It is not weak to perform oral sex on a partner, and she should offer the same gratification in return. It would be rude not to! Oral sex is an act of love. If your partner dislikes oral sex, explain how important it is to fulfill an act of love to create a partner's pleasure. Conversing the salacious desires to your partner will help to build a stronger bond, deeper orgasms, and honor your relationship with newfound respect.

SCENE 3

You and your partner often experiment with foreplay, but it is starting to feel routine. Although she always makes you orgasm through oral sex and masturbation, you crave an extra something to take you to the next thrilling stage of sexuality.

The Problem: A long-term relationship or marriage can reach this typical stage after many satisfactory years. Although you both realize it requires extra oomph, neither of you know how to recreate that magic bedroom chemistry. Perhaps you dabbled with exciting foreplay techniques, but felt it too extraordinarily different to continue, and you both slipped back into the same old sexual routine.

Take Charge: Spontaneity is a useful tool in this instance. Read the chapter on "Hot Foreplay Methods" and experiment with both the scalp massage and buttock squeezing techniques. They both help to create a sexual connection with a partner and stimulate the nerve endings like no other method. Alternatively, experiment with alternative stimulations e.g. food play. Two naked bodies covered in food and/or oil invents two alternate erotic scenes that work to heighten every sense. The fun techniques throughout this guide are guaranteed to build not only a thrilling sex life, but will also build on your levels of patience, control, and desire.

How It Improves Your Sex Life: New sexual techniques that you have not yet experienced will do much more than stimulate each receptive nerve ending in the body. Spontaneous sex will build intensity and invoke the departed passion that once existed in your relationship. Surprise each other with a display of your newfound spontaneous spirit.

SCENE 4

You love sex with your partner, but the only position she will allow for penetration is missionary. She is paranoid about her figure, and believes you view the same. Girl-on-top is never an option, although you wish that she would grow a little self-confidence and display her beautiful figure in exciting positions. You have requested that she dominate you because you crave adventure over basic missionary.

The Problem: She lacks the self-esteem necessary to turn your sex life from average to awesome. She feels comfortable only during missionary position, when your body is covering hers. She has lost all sense of self-worth, and sex between you both is now unexciting. Her insecurity issues drive you insane, but you remain in the relationship to love and support her. Compliments are not enough for paranoid women. They must first learn to love themselves inside and out, and be aware that perfection does not exist; it is a mere illusion conditioned into the masses. Another illusion is that wealth and recognition equals success, and thin equals desirable. In addition, celebrities and models are super-airbrushed before publication. The current beauty projected into the world is another illusion, which you must learn to see through.

Take Charge: Both parties can suffer with bodily confidence issues. Starting today, you must learn to love yourself, including the flaws that magnify through your eyes. Repeat, "I love and approve of myself" four-hundred times per day for thirty days, and read the chapter on "Masturbation" for a great tip that builds on bodily confidence. Everybody is born into the world with the emphasis on beauty equals success and power. We are taught to judge others and ourselves. Rather than judge or see the flaws in others, notice the beauty that is surrounding you daily. Now is the time to make a stand and banish those insecurities forever. Remember your good qualities and allow them to shine through.

How It Improves Your Sex Life: Displaying self-confidence is the sign of a positive, sexy person. At one time or another, everyone has had a little extra flesh on the body, but do not allow it to destroy the once strong relationship you shared with your partner. Men love a confident woman. If you already view yourself as sexy you are in control of your destiny. Enthusiasm is sexy. By choosing to shift your negatives into positives, you take back your power. Experiment with sexual aids during oral sex, domination, rubbing foreplay.

COMMUNICATION

It is a solid feat to maintain a long lasting marriage or relationship, as both require time and effort for long-term success. Communication is important for any relationship, whether platonic or romantic. Do you share your thoughts, feelings, worries, and future hopes with your partner?

If you feel insecure about your body or suffer other doubts, take a leap of faith and communicate all those insecurities to your partner. By halving a problem, the original dilemma will lose its hold, while also bringing you closer to your partner. To maintain a healthy relationship, trust is paramount. Unless your partner has the psychic ability to mind read; it is important to confess your worries and relieve your mind of the current problem affecting your thoughts.

Are you able to confess of the foreplay moves that drive you wild? Do you have a secret fantasy or fetish that you would love to share? Have you told or shown your partner how you like to be touched? If you share the problem, it not only relieves the pressure off your shoulders, but also fills your partner with confidence on so many levels. If you can let down your boundaries and share all your sexual desires with a partner, s/he will feel important and desperate to satisfy you sexually.

Many relationships can suffer through a lack of communication. Stress can easily weave its way into the conscious mind, and some individuals try to create solutions to problems without burdening his/her partner. This may cause tension to rise, which could lead to an angry outburst or manifest problems in other ways. Before you reach the point where stress causes you to react hastily, share the problem with your partner. The advice is likely to reduce your anxiety.

Stress affects most of us daily, plus it can be difficult for most individuals to handle alone. Do not let stress get in the way of your once strong relationship. Refuse to let it exist—state, "Go away" or "Delete" in a loud but calm tone. Alternatively, stand up, stare at the ceiling, and grin for a minute. Knowing you look daft brings out your inner child and could change your mood quickly. If you are conscious of the problem then it will be easier to erase. If you choose to ignore a problem by focusing your thoughts elsewhere, your mind has time to create a solution. When the mind can think clearly, solutions emerge. During a stressful episode, cloudiness can sway any rational decisions.

For married couples—do you remember the vows that were spoken during your ceremony? Always remember that your partner is there to love, honor, and support you through good and bad times. Never try to cope with a problem alone, always share it with a partner or friend.

The Sexual Mind is designed to alleviate stress through the release of natural endorphins—the feel good hormones and pain relievers—and help you to grow closer to your partner. Read the chapter on "Foreplay Fun" and experiment with each method. At first glance, some foreplay moves may seem mediocre, but others may appeal to your curious mind. Sex and orgasms are two fantastic stress busters that cause tension-relieving endorphins to enter the body,

Communication is important; it displays the fact that you trust your partner enough to share the burden. If you find it easy to talk to him/her about your problem, why not disclose your sexual needs—including how you like to be touched intimately. If this is a tough step, first work on building your self-confidence to a level where you can share those kinky thoughts.

Words, thoughts, and fantasies can only be conveyed through conversation and enthusiastic lovemaking. Try not to fake your sexual pleasure. If you require appropriate time to relax your body throughout foreplay, confess this to your partner. I am sure s/he will understand. However, if you fake an orgasm, and your partner discovers this at some point in the future, it could create sexual insecurities in him/her. Instead of allowing it to reach that stage, discuss your issues in an open fashion NOW to create an electrifying sex life.

ANATOMY

THE MALE ANATOMY

The Penis:[3] This is a marvelous organ found within the male genitals. However, it too has received judgments over time. Statements like, "Only a large penis can satisfy a woman," or "Big feet equals a big penis" are age-old myths.

In reality, the average-sized penis is around five and a half inches when erect. Penises come in all shapes and sizes. Some contain a foreskin and others undergo circumcision. The latter reason could be through religion, to feel cleaner, or because his partner is big on hygiene. The size of a penis varies enormously from flaccid to erect, and often by several inches.

Various cultures worldwide believe that a man with a larger than average penis can satisfy a woman far greater than a man with a smaller member. This is another misconception spread by word of mouth, beliefs in culture, and through books.

There are over three billion men worldwide and each has a unique penis. Whether it is the shape, length, width, or the fact that you can reach multi-orgasmic states, no two penises are alike. Caress it with soft strokes during masturbation and let it live out its sexual pleasures.

When flaccid, a man with a smaller than average penis will increase its length by several inches when erect, compared to a man with a larger penis when flaccid, but whose length may only increase by half an inch or less when erect. Penis size is very personal to a man, although confidence is paramount when the aim is to satisfy your partner in the bedroom. A jibe about penis size or inadequate performances can hit a nerve and permanently affect a man's sexual performance.

The penis contains three long narrow cylinders. Inside these cylinders are cavities that fill up with blood during an erection. Normally, they remain limp, but during an erection they fill with blood giving an instant bulge. Human penises are unique in that they do not contain a bone, unlike other mammals that do have a penis bone and additional support during an erection.

Two cylinders rest side by side along the top of the penis; and the third lies on the underside of the penis. Each flexible body is wrapped in a tough coating. In order for the penis to become erect, the wrapper must contain no tears. If it does, the erection may bend rather than point upright. Tears are extremely rare but easily repairable through surgery.

Both semen and urine pass through the urethra, which runs beside the length of the penis. A clever valve system closes off the bladder shaft during ejaculation, and puts an instant stop to urination. The penis tip is filled with nerve endings and extremely sensitive to touch. Some men have a foreskin, which secretes smegma—a fluid to prevent chafing when the penis hardens. This fluid is repetitively smoothed over the area during sex or masturbation.

The Perineum:[4] In men, this highly sensitive area is situated between the scrotum and anus, and in women, between the vulva and anus. On stimulation, it brings forth incredible sensations and can easily heighten an orgasm. It could even turn some individuals multi-orgasmic.

The prostate gland (male g-spot) is located about two inches inside the anus and is the approximate size of a walnut. For a man, stimulation to this hot spot can manifest incredible depths of pleasure. During an orgasm, the male g-spot is often slightly stimulated. Most men may never admit this fact to a partner or they feel content to go through life knowing that an incredibly erotic hot spot is situated inside their anus. A religious belief could set in stating that it is wrong to experiment in this area. However, it is a healthy fascination to experiment with toys, fingers, and lubricants around the sensitive anus. If you feel daring, ask your partner to experiment with his/her finger(s). If you do not prefer direct stimulation by way of a finger, request that your partner rims[5] your ass, or use a vibrating toy. The results will feel exhilarating, shocking, or provide a mixture of both, but I am sure it will feel more erotic than offensive.

For men who have no knowledge of this hot spot, or for those who feel intrigued to experiment further, yet have no idea of what to do, here are some tips:

1. Take a bath or shower to relax the sphincter muscles of the anus. Avoid experimenting when this area is tense—it could create discomfort.
2. Lie down, get comfortable, and spread your legs. If you choose to use a finger as your tool of choice, apply lots of lubricant to the anus and finger(s) beforehand.
3. Gently massage the anus without pushing in a finger or toy. Do not rush—the incredible sensations will come.

4. It may feel both exciting and weird on first entry. However, the urge for a deeper sensation may soon take hold. If using a finger, reach two-inches upwards to feel for the g-spot (a walnut sized fleshy area).

5. During g-spot arousal, your penis could harden and secrete pre-cum. This is normal. The g-spot is highly sensitive, and any direct pressure on this hot spot during intercourse or oral sex could turn the experience even more spectacular.

Become knowledgeable about the male g-spot to enhance your lovemaking. After a bath or shower, take it in turns to rim his/her perineum and anus. You can further heighten the experience by requesting that your partner push in his/her tongue a couple of inches to stimulate the g-spot. This will cause several reactions, which are likely to be intense moans and bodily quivers for the lucky receiver. Women will mould into a Goddess by experimenting with rimming and anal play.

I understand that anal exploration will not suit everyone, but great sex requires commitment and a choice to step out of the ordinary. To achieve incredible depths of pleasure, experiment regularly, and learn to enjoy anal exploration. Will it really kill you to trial and error anal foreplay? If the thought turns you queasy, use a small sex toy and wait for a reaction in your partner. Men can intuitively read if a partner is faking the enjoyment of oral pleasure.

For experimental men who enjoy stimulating their g-spot on a regular basis, buy a butt plug or small vibrator to energize the anus with new sensations. The more toys you experience, the easier you will find it to reach those same levels of ecstasy without having to take illegal drugs to get the same high.

There is nothing dirty or sinful about anal experimentation, especially when the area is clean and toys are washed after use. It is a perfectly healthy and horny way to boost the sex life.

THE FEMALE ANATOMY

The Vagina: During sexual arousal, the vagina lubricates and widens ready for penetration. One of the first psychological signs of arousal in a woman is the secretion of lubricant. This can all take place in less than a minute. When the mind sends a signal to the vagina signaling its arousal just ten to thirty seconds later, tiny beads of fluid form in the vaginal wall to create a glistening cover.

Allow your partner to experience your juices and all pre-sexual worries will subside, forcing fun to shift to the forefront of your mind. Practice with long foreplay sessions to achieve intense orgasms.

The vagina expands like a balloon and the uterus and cervix rise up slowly and back from harms way. During this sexual awakening, the vagina fills with blood and darkens from purplish red to a distinct purple. Throughout oral sex or masturbation, the second stage of arousal excites the orgasmic platform, then during orgasm, the vagina contracts sporadically at 0.8-second intervals three to fifteen times.

Heavily aroused females can experience "super orgasms." These convulsive contractions last from two to four seconds before reducing to the normal 0.8-second spasms. In the final stage and after climax, the orgasmic platform drains the blood, the vaginal opening expands, and the swollen inner vagina decreases in size back to its primary stage. The usual color returns in ten to fifteen minutes as it relaxes and returns to normal.

The Female G-Spot: Whether this hot spot is myth or fiction, why not find out for yourself. Experts state that the female g-spot—full of rich nerve endings, is situated one to two inches inside the front of the vaginal wall. If you have penetrated this hot spot with a finger through foreplay, it feels fleshy—very similar to the male g-spot. Listen to your own body and experiment. Masturbation and sexual relations with another will help you to reinstate the wondrous changes that take place in the body during sexual arousal and intercourse.

The best positions to stimulate this hot spot are doggy style[6] and knees on shoulder position during missionary. It can cause varied reactions in women; some may find it comfortable and exciting, whereas it may feel too deep and uncomfortable for others. It may turn other women multi-orgasmic.

In 1950, Ernst Grafenberg, M.D., a gynecologist and obstetrician wrote an article concluding that a small area situated in the upper vagina can produce orgasms without clitoral stimulation, hence the name Grafenberg spot or g-spot.[7] Since the discovery of the g-spot in the 50s, millions of women have experienced the pleasures of this hot spot, including myself.

Other women believe the female g-spot is a myth because they feel nothing spectacular during penetration. Every woman is different. What one woman may experience as nothing spectacular could satisfy another woman to incredible heights. Do not give up on the pleasures of this hot spot. Women are born with an incredible number of nerve endings in the genitals. Now is the time to take charge of your body and experiment with toys, lubricants, and diverse sexual positions.

Female Ejaculation: When a woman orgasms, the vagina naturally secretes lubrication. Squirting is another form of female ejaculation—fluid also secreted from the urethra. Stimulation of the g-spot can feel a lot like urination before ejaculation occurs. However, after orgasm, many women secrete droplets or gush a wave of lubrication during and after orgasm. This can trigger a strong urge to urinate. This fluid is produced by the Skene's gland (the female prostate); a group of ducts situated beside the entrance of the urethra. Research has shown that this liquid does not contain urine, but very similar components like those secreted from the male g-spot.

Skeptics believe that no such female g-spot exists, and the ejaculation secreted from the urethra is very much like urine.[8] I have ejaculated from the urethra during masturbation, and this is not urine. During clitoral stimulation or passionate kisses, ejaculation can also secrete from the vagina in very aroused women.

The Clitoris: This is a smart little hot spot full of rich nerve endings. If you are female, consider yourself lucky! Unlike a multi-functional penis that allows for urination, sexual pleasure, and ejaculation, the purpose of the clitoris is to provide only orgasmic pleasure. Certain sexual positions may not always stimulate the clitoris, but it is possible to work this hot spot into the sexual equation with careful foreplay. Toys are fun to use alone or with a partner. Stroke your clitoris while sat on top of him to effortlessly excite his penis.

Throughout foreplay, a penis rubbed over the clitoris can feel very pleasurable for many women. It drives me nuts! If you want to regain your feminine power, do not allow your partner to penetrate you until you achieve a real orgasm. Whether it takes a couple of minutes or several hours, remember to focus on your pleasure. Never fake it.

The penis is sensitive to touch after orgasm, and so too is the clitoris. They look very similar when viewed internally, although the clitoris is hidden by the clitoral hood, and only pops out of its shell during arousal. Unbelievably, the length of the clitoris is four inches—the exact length of an average sized flaccid penis. The rest of the organ is hidden from sight, and the clitoris grows erect filling with blood during arousal, changing from its normal dark red to a distinguished purple. In some women, the clitoris may look larger and easily perceivable, but in others, it slips away from sight under the protective clitoral hood.

Many women need only slight stimulation on the clitoris to reach arousal and orgasm. In other women, the clitoris requires constant attention to reach sexual ecstasy. Masturbation is a useful foreplay move to add to any lovemaking session. Try solo masturbation alone, or invite your partner into the equation and masturbate together. Listen to your body. Experiment with positions that make it easier for your partner to stroke your clitoris, e.g. doggy style, girl-on-top, or try rubbing foreplay before full penetration.

If masturbation is foreign, or you believe it to be shameful, try to remember who first put that thought into your subconscious mind. I believe that we should all seek ways to expand the powerful mind and enjoy the free pleasures that are available. Orgasms, masturbation, and sex are three of the infinite joys we can experience right now. Do you choose to experience this freedom or ignore your sexual urges because another person told you it was wrong? If you want to experience sexual liberty, strip off your clothes, stroke your clitoris to a fulfilling orgasm, and tighten the vagina in the process.

Every orgasm feels astonishingly different. Some can last longer or feel more powerful than previous orgasms. However, they are also dependent on how aroused you feel during the process. Other orgasms may feel like a quick release of tension, yet it is possible to adjust your mindset to enjoy any sexual experience. You can build an orgasm that feels breathtaking through the simple focus of your sexual thoughts on every pleasurable move.

Experiment: If you have no idea where your g-spot resides, now is the time to experiment and find it. Remain seated upright when feeling for this fleshy hot spot. Insert a toy or finger(s) and then reach about two inches into the upper front of the vaginal wall. The first thing you will experience during stimulation of the g-spot is the urgent need to urinate. If you empty the bladder beforehand, there is no need to worry. The internal area will feel swollen and lumpy, but every woman is different. It may be situated a little higher in the upper front wall of the vagina in some women.

The ideal sexual positions to stimulate the female g-spot are deep penetrative positions like reverse cowgirl, doggy style, or girl-on-top. It is possible to be in any position during clitoral stimulation, although it will require concentration to reach your peak.

If masturbation feels strange, lie down in a comfortable position and breathe deeply to relax the body. Allow your mind to wander into fantasyland. If this takes five minutes or fifty minutes, do not let time distract from your feeling of inner peace. Do you feel a sudden twitch in your vagina when your mind delves deeper into the fantasy, or perhaps the horny thoughts turn you juicier than normal?

If you struggle to grow excited, try to think of something out of the ordinary that you would never contemplate in reality, e.g. dressing in rubber and letting your partner cover you in oil, while he rubs his naked body over your oily rubber clad body.

Rub the clitoris slowly and experiment with varied finger pressures. If you prefer to use a toy, let a vibrating dildo work its magic. Some women find it easier to stimulate their clitoris if the hood is pulled back slightly. Focus only on the pleasure in your mind, and remain patient until you reach the brink of ecstasy.

YOUR SEXUAL POWER

ATTRACTION AND SCENTS

There are over six billion humans worldwide, and besides identical twins, no two people look the same. I am glad about the latter; the world would be a very boring place otherwise. Variety is the spice of life. What one-person views as attractive another may deem the opposite. An example of this would be a man who prefers a plain but confident woman beside an insecure stunning female. Although most of the men would opt for the stunning woman as a "trophy bird," deep down most men will feel strangely attracted to the confident, plainer girl. Her confidence reigns high above judgments from others, and bitchy comments will not affect her subconsciously.

Confidence is sexy regardless of attractiveness. Some men like to date only high maintenance women who take hours to get ready for a date. These egotistical women often think they are God's gift and only date rich men to wine and dine them. Other men enjoy dating down-to-earth women who they can relax and have a laugh with.

Who you choose to date states a lot about how you view yourself. If you date or attract only game players, you may be displaying insecurity or self-conscious issues because you feel hopeless and unworthy inside. The subconscious mind is extremely powerful, but it is straightforward to change your mindset through various techniques, e.g. hypnosis, meditation, positive affirmations, and/or brainwave entrainment. Always value yourself. If you take pride in your appearance and state that you are worthy of a loving partner, be patient, visualize your happiness, and trust the Universe.

Chemistry is of prime importance during the initial stages of attraction, but it need not only relate to sex either. Friendship equals chemistry, a mental connection between long-distance partners equals chemistry, and good communication between couples equals chemistry. Let your pheromones guide you to interesting people and potential prey. Always listen to your intuition—the inner voice from your Higher Self that is often ignored.

If you meet a potential partner, and the first kiss is good, agree to a date with him/her. If the first kiss does not make your heart flutter, your instinctive pheromones may be indicating that you are not a sexually compatible match with him/her. The first kiss can be extremely important to most individuals; so let your pheromones intuitively guide you toward the perfect partner.

Is a Partner Required to Feel Loved? Some individuals crave a partner to feel desired and loved. True love cannot be forced. The more you try to force love into your life, the more you may find yourself hopping out of one dead-end relationship into the next, experiencing more heartache along the way. The men/women who go round in circles of heartbreak will only attract true love if s/he first develops a relationship with the self. When you radiate inner peace and love inward, you send out a vibration to the Universe that states, "I'm ready for love."

Attracting true love is based on the thoughts you think about consciously. The Law of Attraction gives you exactly what you think about consciously or unconsciously. If you constantly tell yourself that you are unworthy of a loving partner, then you will attract more partners who will give you reason to doubt yourself. Be careful what you wish for, especially when you desire love.

What you must first understand about love is that it will not manifest in your life unless you build a relationship with yourself first. Buy well fitting clothes, masturbate and embrace your solo orgasms, eat nutritious food, exercise regularly, and meditate to clear the mind. Give yourself at least an hour of "me time" each day.

Society has not helped in the quest for love. With an abundance of dating sites, and the celebrity world hopping in and out of relationships with each other, we are taught that the single life is desperate, when this is so far from the truth. The single life is a fun time, which allows you to regain independence. Spending time alone with the self teaches you to look at your current life and make a list of what you view as attractive in your perfect partner. It is brave and mature to move away from a static relationship. If you are in a stale partnership, step out of the picture and become the true character that others describe you to be. You do not have to settle for second best or remain in a limited relationship. Often it is better to go it alone.

Do your friends and family compliment your hairstyle, personality, smile, or fashion sense? Do you accept those compliments or doubt them because of a deeper insecurity you have yet to acknowledge? I attract an abundance of compliments about my positive personality and style, and I accept these with gratitude. I send out love and happiness to the Universe and it returns to me daily to keep me on the high vibration of love. Do not underestimate the power of positive thought and kindness toward others.

Compliments work on boosting the ego, but it is better to accept and state your gratitude to the Universe to sustain a high vibration. It is difficult to alter the mindset to positive, but it is possible with determination. Just as an individual can decide to quit smoking through will power, it is possible to alter the mindset with positive affirmations, meditation, hypnosis, or even brainwave entrainment. Only when you love and accept yourself will your inner soul attract to you a loving partner who is a magnet of your qualities.

If you act out of desperation to meet a partner, you may attract the same. However, if you decide to use the Law of Attraction to manifest your perfect partner, you must be willing to plant the seed (vision and thought) with the Universe, visualize the outcome, and remain patient without doubt. If a shred of uncertainty prevails, the Universe will slow down or destroy your projection. Faith is always a requirement with the Law of Attraction.

A very powerful method that can be used to attract love is to imagine you have already met your dream partner, and plan your life ahead of the manifestation. As soon as you have planted your seed with the abundant Universe, be grateful that your request has already been fulfilled, and NEVER question when or how you will meet him/her. Surrender to what will be, and the Universe will bless you in the most magical of ways.

Any lack-based thoughts, such as, "I am never going to find true love," will not help to manifest your desire. However, if you stop the negative thoughts and alter them into positive affirmations e.g., "True love is on its way to me," you can strengthen your vision. Describe your future partner—be very descriptive (eyes, hair, personality, height, traits, attractiveness, tattoos etc), detach your thoughts, and return to your daily duties. The Universe is already at work lining up the right day and time for you to meet him/her.

Remember the positive statement, "Good things come to those who wait." The Law of Attraction works in that exact way. Pessimism or doubt will slow down your manifestation, or too much negativity can affect the flow of abundance into your life. However, if you believe in your vision and detach your thoughts, your dream WILL manifest. The Law of Attraction is one of the many spiritual laws of the Universe.[9]

Some men/women cope well alone, but other individuals find it extremely difficult or downright depressing to be without a partner long-term. I continue to watch some of my friends jump in and out of one unfulfilling relationships to the next in the space of only weeks/months. It rarely works out over the long-term, because s/he is on the lookout for someone better.

Conscious thoughts that include this focus will not convey true happiness either. If you are unfulfilled with a partner and seek "someone better," the Universe will continue to supply you with unsatisfying partners who make you think exactly that way. Although it can take time for certain individuals to realize that true love cannot be forced, until the point of self-realization, s/he will continue down the road of destruction, wasting more precious time and energy on unsuitable partners.

Quite often after a relationship ends badly, desperate singletons may seek another partner to build a fulfilling relationship with. However, this may not be a great match, and could even end in more heartbreak. The thought of being single or the constant pressure to be with somebody through judgmental friends and family can feel terrifying for an individual whose only aim in life is to fall in love.

In the past, I felt exactly this way. I attracted game playing assholes who disrespected me and made me feel small. However, I had not yet developed a relationship with myself, nor did I love myself unconditionally. I criticized myself constantly for being unable to keep a man. After several years of spending time alone, I cannot get enough of my own company. Although true love is beautiful to find, it is also difficult to find a true-life partner who supports your life choices and feels your every emotion.

Life is too short to spend a quarter of your life in and out of dead-end relationships, which further drains the body of precious energy. At the beginning of a relationship, every moment feels exciting and nothing feels weird or out of place. After several months or years with that person, unbeknown problems could start to manifest. Do you ignore them or believe in a long-term future with your beloved? What do your instincts state? If it states the obvious—things are not meant to be—why choose to put your mental and physical body through a dreary relationship that will only lead to more unhappiness and doubt?

Choose to incorporate meditation into your daily life, make new friends, and build a healthy social life with likeminded individuals. The urgent desire to seek a partner will diminish, and the next time you meet a potential partner, s/he could be the complete opposite of whom you normally date. Instinctively, you know that the relationship will build into something beautiful because you did not blow out "desperate" vibes.

No doubt you have heard the expression, "When you stop looking for love, it will find you?" Both parties find it easy to smell a desperate vibe from a mile away. If you have never spent time alone to develop a relationship with the self or been aware that you hop in and out of one fruitless relationship to the next, it would be extremely rare to find a true-life partner.

Individuals who seek a partner in desperation will subconsciously demonstrate this through his/her body language. An individual who is constantly on the lookout for a partner, but also judging of others is insecure and likely to attract the same qualities in a partner. Subconsciously, s/he has no idea of the desperate vibes sent out through energetic vibrations, but it is a deeper insecurity that s/he must first admit to the self as regards to the need for a partner to feel happy. It may be difficult to admit this fact, but self-love is the main criteria to work on in order to meet a well-matched partner. One person who relies heavily on another forms attachment and conditional love, which could turn a relationship difficult.

The aim of a successful relationship is to love another unconditionally. Detach yourself from a partner, but send out love by wishing him/her well. Conditional love is easy to spot, e.g. jealousy of another, reliance on another person for happiness, and high expectations during a relationship or marriage.

To attract a partner, first stop looking outside of yourself, and enjoy the current moment. Love yourself unconditionally, rely on yourself—never another, and stop searching for love as a way to feel whole. If looks are one of the main components you seek in a partner, try to let down your boundaries and date an individual who is the complete opposite of your usual "type." Good looks will always fade, but personality remains timeless.

Seven years of being alone taught me that I am not worthless. I dated insufficient losers who mentally abused me. For many years, I suffered with heavy trust issues and deemed myself unworthy of ever finding true love. I experimented sexually and believed no man would take on my open sexuality or past conquests. However, it can happen and it did happen to me. I met a special man in the most unusual of ways. He encouraged me to write this book and has never judged my past. A true-life partner would never judge you; only inspire you to build on your talents. We are no longer together, but I forgive his mistakes. Keith was not the right man for me, and I think we both knew that deep down, hence the Universe working its magic to break us apart.

Attraction: We pass hundreds, perhaps thousands of people per day throughout our daily lives. How many of those individuals do you glance at twice? The answer could be many. It is natural to look at and desire a member of the opposite sex, or the same sex if homosexual.

Both men/women are highly visible creatures. Men can walk around with their tops off, and if his body is well defined, women admire his confidence from afar. Daydreaming is a healthy fascination and pumps the mind with dozens of sexy images. Loving couples can look at and fancy other people, except s/he does not act upon those carnal fantasies. It feels naughty to think about sex during the day, especially in a meeting at work, and I find it fascinating that no one else can read our thoughts. If a machine or person existed to read our thoughts, free will would no longer exist.

Luckily, you do not have to feel on edge or warrant a spank from a partner for visualizing about sex with another person. The human mind is a secret computer full of knowledge, and I hope you agree that it is better to remain that way.

It is a healthy fascination to find other individuals (other than your partner) attractive. This does not count as infidelity, nor should you feel guilty. Sight is a wonderful sense for lucky souls, but it is unfortunate for individuals who are unable to see through illness, disability, or injury. A "sixth sense" may develop in these individuals, or one or more of his/her original four senses could heighten or develop into a psychic power.

Another important factor with attraction are the initial "magical pheromones" that force you to glance at another without knowing why. His/her "look" gripped your attention, so the curiosity to find out more about him/her takes control, and butterflies enter the tummy. Only during an initial conversation will you find out if you *do* share common interests with him/her.

The first couple of minutes of a conversation have the most importance over any other stage of a relationship. This is because during those first few seconds or minutes, you make a decision on whether s/he is interesting enough to want to get to know further. For example, does s/he mirror your body language, make eye contact when you speak and nod in agreement, or have dilated pupils? These are positive signs of attraction. If s/he subconsciously displays these strong body language signals, the question you must now ask yourself is, do you feel the same way?

Good conversation with a member of the opposite sex or same sex holds more importance over looks. With confidence often comes arrogance and huge egos, but these individuals are often easy to spot in a crowded room. His/her clothes and jewelry may be over the top, and s/he may act brash around others. It is quite rare to find a naturally confident individual who exhibits no egotistical side. When you do meet a confident person, watch him/her work the crowd and use personality to magnetically attract others.

Have you ever kissed someone whom you found attractive, only to discover that you felt no sexual chemistry with him/her? It could be that your chemical DNA does not match his/hers. Pheromones are invisible hormones that seek out a reciprocal partner in order to mate healthy children. If two people enter a relationship without chemistry, yet remain together anyway; it may be impossible to build mutual attraction and love. It is better to develop a loving relationship with the self, wait patiently, and let cupid play its part.

When you meet the right person, and the conversation flows magically, it is very likely that his/her pupils will dilate. Genuine smiles and flirtatious glances that last longer than two seconds is another positive sign. If s/he holds your gaze and smiles, there is a genuine attraction. When you communicate, does s/he lean in closer as you talk so that your faces almost brush together? This is also a very positive sign. What about an excuse to touch you, perhaps a playful slap on the hand, or purposely brushing a hand against the clothes? If yes, this is a subconscious display of attraction toward you.

Mirroring body language is an important sign of attraction, especially if you remain alert and carefully spot his/her "moves." The pupils of drug takers also enlarge, but I am sure you can distinguish a drug user over an individual who finds your sexual aura magnetic.

Sexual Scents: Pheromones are found in both men/women through the secretion of smegma. Natural pheromones also emit from urine and perspiration. If you feel attracted to another during a workout at the gym, your pheromones[10] are in charge and trying to seek a partner of the same caliber.

The perfume and pharmaceutical industries are worth billions. The latter take advantage of lonely individuals who seek love and affection. Advertisements, usually by way of genius marketing online, then state that an expensive synthetic pheromone spray will attract a compatible mate. Androstenol, a natural pheromone secreted by men/women, is added to pheromone sprays. Although these scents are potent, do not forget the fact that your body contains natural pheromones—odorless scents that play cupid to attract a compatible partner. Why do you feel that they are not working on your behalf? They work 24/7 on attraction, but if you choose to cover up your pheromones with perfumes, aftershaves, scented face and body creams, and deodorants, the concentration of essential oils mixed with alcohol covers your natural scent.[11]

A huge population of the world use perfumes, aftershaves, or synthetic pheromone sprays to "heighten" his/her attraction to others, but love and attraction cannot create a synchronistic partnership. Perfumes and aftershaves contain a high degree of essential oils mixed into an alcohol base, which "attract" a member of the opposite or same sex. In reality, it feels like your "pheromones" are at work, but these are synthetic scents.[12] A high proportion of pheromone or sex sprays, however, do contain real pheromones, and scientific studies state that they work, but are they necessary? I have attracted some great sexual partners by going au natural, but could you? I do wear perfumes when the mood strikes, although my favorite has been discontinued.

Everyone is born with his/her own unique, enticing scent. Why would you want to cover this with expensive perfumes/aftershaves/deodorants? If you believe that synthetic fragrances enhance your natural pheromones, think again! If the perfume industry let you in on this secret, sales would gradually decline. I am a truth seeker, and I only want to spread this information to others.

Natural pheromones are secreted through perspiration, urine, and sexual fluids. Perspiration is odorless, but only when bacteria breeds through stress does bad odor become distinctive. Are you willing to experiment with your own natural pheromones to observe the results they bring? Before a night out, spray on your favorite perfume or aftershave and note the results of whom you attract? Are you sexually compatible through sex, foreplay, and passionate kisses? Alternatively, why not go au natural with a dab of your natural lubricant on the pulse points of the body, ideally after a bath or shower. Note the results. I hope that it provides an insight into how powerful your scent can attract a sexually compatible partner.

Interesting Pheromone Facts: Men secrete a chemical pheromone through their natural body odor, but women can only absorb this during an intimate encounter. This pheromone works like magic to make a woman sexually healthy. Women who have sex just once a week could find their menstrual cycles normalize, and they become more fertile than women who practice celibacy or irregular sex.

Women secrete a pheromone called menstrual synchrony, which is the reason why a group of women who live together often start their menstrual cycles together, or a couple of days apart. Female pheromones can also wander across a room to attract a partner, whereas men must have intimate contact with a woman for his pheromones to take effect.[13]

After orgasm, women secrete another hormone, oxytocin, which forms a bond with a partner. While women are often loving and affection toward a partner after sex and orgasm, men are far less empathetic, which can be frustrating for women.

Dab your natural pheromones on pulse points, e.g. wrists, back of the ears, nape of the neck, inside of elbows, around the belly button, and backs of the knees. Also, follow these simple body language tips:

- **Smile**: This bold gesture displays confidence toward a stranger. A fake smile is easily distinguishable through two facial gestures, (1) the face becomes asymmetrical, and (2) the eyes do not move. A natural smile highlights the lines around the eyes, and the face displays symmetry.

- **Make Eye Contact**: After capturing the attention of an admirer, try this move. Catch his/her eye, look away, then glance back and try to hold his/her stare for a full two seconds. If you must, count the seconds in your head silently. If you stare longer than the initial two seconds, you could cause offense. If s/he looks a little embarrassed, but gazes away then back toward you, there is a definite attraction.

- **Use Gloss/Lipstick**: Highlight your lips with a bold colored lipstick or shiny gloss after capturing the attention of your admirer. Clear gloss is always easy to apply without a mirror and will instantly grip his attention onto your pout. Another flirty move is to lick your lips to draw further attention to your pout. Your admirer is likely to be fantasizing about a first kiss, and some kinky men will be imagining your lips elsewhere.

- **Hands In The Pocket**: Used by men, this gesture displays confidence and self-assurance.

- **Hair Twirling**: This is a powerful move for any woman to try on a potential admirer, especially after you have made intensive eye contact with him. Hair twirling draws his attention to the elegant kissable neck, plus it is a known flirtatious move.

- **Display a Cheeky Side**: Wink at your admirer, or if you feel confident, pinch the buttocks to capture his/her attention. Only try this move if you have received a positive signal from your admirer, e.g. the two-second stare or a genuine smile. In some circumstances, and only if you believe it will not cause offense, compliment him/her in a sexually provocative manner. As an example, one of my ex-boyfriends approached me in a nightclub to state how hard he became while watching me dance. I loved the compliment, and we dated for several months. This move may cause offense to many women, but it is a massive ego boost for open-minded women.

- **Have Fun**: The best thing you can do to attract a partner is to love your own company. Show the world that you do not need a partner to display confidence and happiness. This will raise your vibration to magnetic. When you are out with your friends, study the room for men/women who intrigue you. Watch his/her body language. A "desperate vibe" is evident, so keep that in mind when you are on the lookout for potential prey. On a night out with friends, move onto the dance floor or chat with strangers to make new friends. Act comfortable in your own company and compliment others. Energy acts like a magnet—what you give out will return to you.

- **Alcohol**: Get a little tipsy, but remain aware of your surroundings. Drink spiking still occurs, so never let your drink out of your sight. Many drugs cause blackouts, which makes it easy for the "spiker" to commit a sexual act without your content. Fruit or minty breath is sexy; beer breath is not.

- **Smoking**: The sweet stench of smoke masks all scents on the body, including perfumes, aftershaves, scented body cream, and natural pheromones. There is nothing positive about smoking. It ages the skin, yellows the teeth, causes heart disease, cancer(s), and is the main cause of breathing and circulatory problems. Quit smoking today and look forward to better health, improved lung function, whiter teeth, sweeter breath, and improved taste buds.

- **Dress For Yourself**: If you follow the current fashion trends, you may notice that you look more coordinated than out of place. Although fashion is exciting, wearing the same trend is nothing unique. Look at your wardrobe. Do you have an eccentric item of clothing that is often admired by another? Add an original item of clothing to your wardrobe and it may grab the attention of someone likeminded. Some men choose to make a bold statement by painting their nails black or using black eyeliner. Alternatively, a man can wow the crowd with a bright stylish shirt.

- **Be Genuine**: Do not put on a front or act the goat[14] to get other people to like you. Be genuine and allow your personality to shine through. Not everyone "gets me," although I just believe it to be a matter of different vibrations. The law of attraction—like attracts like, works constantly to give you what you focus upon. If you choose to send out a negative or lack vibration, you will receive more situations to feel negative for, including unhelpful people and situations. Alternatively, if you choose to send out positive thoughts through love and gratitude, you will attract likeminded individuals who think similarly.

A Natural Scrub To Entice: Perfumes and aftershaves contain a variety of essential oils, which smell divine when blended to the perfect combination. Mixed with carrier oils, including sweet almond or jojoba, essential oils manipulate the nervous system in positive ways. However, in heavily scented products e.g. perfumes and aftershaves, essential oils are added to an alcohol base. Theoretically, adding unnatural scent to your body masks the pheromones, immobilizing their natural pulling power.

Half of the perfumes I use are now discontinued, and I am not attracted to most of the floral scents available today. I make my own body scrubs with natural ingredients, which helps my body to smell fresh, unique, and sexy. Because the ingredients in this scrub are edible, they work to enhance your natural powers of seduction. Smother your body in this scrub during a bath or shower, and you will smell luscious wherever you walk. Whenever I use this scrub I receive fantastic compliments.

Each 50g tub makes enough scrub to use three times on the whole body. This also works out a lot cheaper than shop bought scrubs, which contain ingredients to give the product a longer shelf life. Most scrubs contain preservatives, which can be harsh on sensitive skins. As the skin is the largest breathable organ in the body, all harmful chemicals and toxins in skincare products[15] are absorbed. Start to use homemade products on your body, and help the environment in the process.

Once opened, keep this homemade scrub in the fridge and use within one month. The ingredients for this natural scrub are easy to find in a health food shop or online. 100g of Shea butter and coconut oil will be enough to make four tubs of scrub.

Natural Ingredients
<ul><li>Medium sized plastic tub (50ml)</li><li>100g brown or white sugar (or sea salt if preferred)</li><li>Two tablespoons of Shea butter</li><li>Spoon of instant coffee (great for cellulite)</li><li>Two tablespoons of coconut oil</li></ul>

Method

1. Measure the sugar ready to mix with the Shea butter and coconut oil and then put to one side. To make a finer scrub, use caster sugar. Natural cane sugar is an effective scrub, but the larger granules could feel harsh and abrasive on very sensitive skin.

2. Add two tablespoons of solidified coconut oil to the plastic tub and mix well. For best results, melt the coconut oil before adding to the tub. Add to the microwave for five seconds to melt the oil, or use a small sauccpan and heat on the hob.

3. Add the sugar/sea salt and/or caster sugar to the tub and mix well into the coconut oil. There should be an oily residue. This added moisturizer, when used as a scrub, nourishes the epidermis—the external layer of the skin. When you use this scrub in the bath or shower, the coconut oil can leave an oily residue in the bath or shower, so be careful not to slip and injure yourself.

4. Add two tablespoons of Shea butter to the pot and mix well with the coconut/sugar consistency until it forms a smooth paste.

5. Cellulite sufferers can add a teaspoon of instant coffee to the potion, or dilute it in a little water before adding to the scrub. When applied externally, coffee releases fluid tension and energizes every cell in the body. Cellulite is a simple accumulation of excess fluid settling under the fatty deposits in the skin, giving the dreaded dimpled effect. Coffee also scents the skin deliciously.

This scrub is gentle enough to use daily, or use it twice weekly for best results. With its abundance of natural ingredients, which scent the body deliciously and enhance your natural pheromones, this energizing scrub will gather compliments. The scrub is free of harsh preservatives—perfect for sensitive skins.

The same sized tub of scrub purchased in a shop is likely to cost double, or through a well-known skincare brand, four times as much. Shea butter costs on average $6.50 (£4.00) per 100ml pot, and coconut oil on average $12.00 (£7.50) per 250g pot. Plastic tubs are available to buy in bulk or separately via online retailers.

The divine scent from the natural ingredients in this scrub leaves your skin kissably soft and lightly scented. When mixed together, Shea butter, coconut oil, sugar, and coffee leave your body smelling fresh, sexy, and enhance your natural powers of attraction.

Make Your Own Natural Perfume: Essential oils work effectively on the nervous system, when mixed with carrier oils. This easy to make natural perfume will enhance your natural pheromones, plus essential oils work positively in other ways. Many shop bought perfumes use vanilla essential oil as the base note, but vanilla essential oil smells nothing like the vanilla essence contained in candles or air fresheners. Vanilla essential oil is also a natural known aphrodisiac.

Natural Ingredients
▪ Small tub or an old perfume bottle
▪ Lemon essential oil
▪ Vanilla essential oil
▪ Teaspoon of olive oil (or use more depending on size of bottle/tub)
Method
1. Add the olive oil to the perfume bottle or small tub. If the container is larger, use more oil.
2. Add four drops of vanilla essential oil to the tub or bottle.
3. Add four drops of lemon essential oil to the tub or bottle.
4. Add the lid, and shake the container thoroughly.
5. Apply to pulse points e.g. wrists, nape of the neck, inside elbows, backs of knees etc.

Benefits of Home Made Perfume

- Essential oils used neat or mixed in carrier oils are potent and benefit the body. A little goes a long way with essential oils. Just one drop of this homemade perfume is enough to cover two pulse points, and the scent will last far longer than expensive designer perfumes.

- Alcohol absorbs the potency of essential oils and is drying to the skin. Use jojoba or sweet almond carrier oils as the base for essential oil, and allow the beneficial oils to penetrate the deepest layers of the skin—the dermis.

- As a bonus, essential oils benefit the nervous system, treating everything from acne and hay fever to athlete's foot and toothache. If perfumes/aftershaves were a known cure for psoriasis or other skin ailments, the news would be worldwide. Sadly, perfumes/aftershaves do not benefit the health of mankind. They exist only to create massive profits.

Benefits of Lemon Essential Oil[16]

- It calms the mind, therefore reducing stress, anxiety, and other problems that arise from nervous tension.
- The scent of lemon is uplifting and works effectively to remove negative entities from the human energy field.
- Lemon essential oil trains the mind to become alert and boosts concentration. As a stimulant, it boosts energy levels, but also acts as a sedative for insomniacs.
- When used regularly, lemon essential oil elevates the white blood cell count in the body, and also improves circulation.

Benefits of Vanilla Essential Oil[17]

- It contains aphrodisiac properties, plus vanilla essential oil works on the mind, body, and spirit to combat depression, relax the body, boost the immune system—by neutralizing free radicals, and acts as a sedative during stressful periods.
- Vanilla essential oil smells overwhelmingly different from vanilla scented air-fresheners. Both vanilla scented foods and fragrances do not use natural essential oil of vanilla, but components derived from hydrocarbons. This does uplift the spirit, but natural essential oil of vanilla contains far more benefits.
- Vanilla essential oil stimulates testosterone in men and estrogen in women, and it also helps sufferers of impotence and frigidity. Dot vanilla on your body (mixed with carrier oil), and your depression or anxiety will alleviate. Vanilla essential oil enhances the mood, plus it contains natural sedative properties.
- It is evident that both lemon and vanilla essential oils, when mixed together, calm the body and mind.

FANTASIES AND FETISHES

Have you ever set your mind free to wander into fantasy? During a daydream, the mind enters a theta state[18] and its creativity enhances. In the theta state, inspiration strikes, long-forgotten memories return, and the mind encounters flashes of dreamlike imagery.

Do you daydream of a hot fantasy on a daily basis? Daydreams invoke the creative part of the mind and are wonderful to employ with sexual experimentation and/or fantasies/fetishes. Think of a fantasy[19] or fetish to unleash your salacious desires. If the fantasy does not feature your partner, do not feel guilty. If your partner has no idea of the images surpassing your sexual mind, do not give it a second thought. Fantasies are natural, healthy, and stimulate the mind into arousal. Fetishes utilize an image or specific item to first create arousal in the mind. The usual fetishes include rubber, BDSM, and stockings/suspenders.

Fantasies are fictional—if you choose to keep them imaginary, but other fantasies are better acted out in reality. However, it is not always beneficial to act upon a fantasy, especially if it later causes a rift in your relationship. On the other hand, excitement often seizes the rational part of the mind. As an example, most men fantasize of a lesbian encounter. To view your partner kissing another female during a threesome enhances this fantasy, turning her into a Goddess.

There are hundreds of fantasies, including domination, group sex and bondage. Usual fetishes include stockings/suspenders, leather boots, latex, and the notorious foot fetish. However, there are other less pronounced fetishes, including the pain of a tattoo, asphyxiation, sniffing worn panties, and WAM[20]. I believe there is a website out there for every type of fetish.

A fantasy acted out in reality may cause a diverse reaction between couples. Some can strengthen or weaken a relationship. Threesomes sound hot, yet they require one hundred percent trust between partners to guarantee success. If you share a strong bond with your partner, group sex could benefit your relationship. However, if you would rather not act out a specific fantasy, but you do so anyway to please a partner, the decision could haunt you at some point in the future. Be respectful toward your mind and body, whichever decision you decide upon.

If the thought of a threesome stimulates your genitals, I would request that you discuss it in depth with your partner beforehand. If you have no doubt, experiment with a threesome as a 'one-off'. Possible questions you could ask yourself include, "will group sex strengthen our relationship," or "will group sex destroy our future?" Be honest while answering these questions, and listen to your instincts.

Sexually adventurous couples may have lingering thoughts of a kinky threesome encounter, which can add instant fireworks and transform a relationship, if you both share a similar mindset. Honesty is the best policy, especially if you agree to the deed but your heart does not speak the truth.

Some sexual fantasies border unusual, or even illegal. Rape or incest is a regular fantasy for some women, but fantasizing of this scene does not signify that she wants to have sex with a family member, or desires to be raped. These particular fantasies could signify a subconscious need to be dominated by a partner. The mind is the hottest erogenous zone in the body. Without it, sex becomes lack luster.

Individuals with a belief that fantasy, masturbation, and erotic thoughts cause embarrassment or guilt could suffer with Hypoactive Desire Disorder—lack of sexual interest. Specialist therapists teach sexually disinterested individuals to open the mind to fantasize during a sexual encounter.

The power of the mind makes it easy to reach orgasm. Tap into this hot erogenous zone by adding fantasy to any sexual encounter. Alternatively, use a fetish item, e.g. rubber, to see how it affects your mind and body during sex or masturbation. This is testimony to the potency of the fertile mind when charged with erotic thoughts.

Fantasy can take place whenever you allow your mind to wander. It is creative and naughty, especially if you allow your sexual mind to focus on rude thoughts at work. Have you tried to climax without a sexual thought or image? It is almost impossible! Imagine a hot fantasy starring your partner, or visualize a sexy stranger. Let your mind create emotion in your body, and focus on how you would turn on him/her in the fantasy. If you feel tension in your genitals, your creative fantasy has worked its magic.

When the mind and genitals synchronize to create arousal, it invokes a horny side creating sexual tension—perfect to use in a spicy sexual encounter. An example of this would be a woman who fantasizes of performing oral sex on her best female friend, yet in reality, she is one hundred percent heterosexual. However, after a wet dream or solo sex, if the image remains clear in her consciousness, it has already triggered the extra sensory part of her mind. This creates sexual prowess and could turn her into an experimental minx in the bedroom.

Try to think out of the box, even if it seems weird or dirty at the time. Image the fantasy in detail to get your juices flowing. Build up the fantasy and drive yourself into a frenzied state before pouncing on your partner. Fantasy is popular because it encourages the mind to expand.

In between fantasy, if you suddenly become curious about homosexuality, do not freak! In no way does this mean that you want to act upon those sexual preferences; it is your curious mind at work. A fantasy can become reality, but most individuals are not ready to share the inner workings of the human mind with a partner. However inhibitions can disappear after alcohol, and a couple may feel open minded enough to share those fantasies, just not act upon them.

Other surreal fantasies like bestiality[21] or incest are nothing extraordinary, but they are scenes you would not act upon in reality. Most importantly, if a strange image slips into your mind triggering your arousal, do not feel guilty or think you have turned into a "weirdo." If you feel embarrassed or ashamed, push the fantasy to one side and focus on something you *do* enjoy. The mind is flooded with over forty thousand thoughts daily. Strange thoughts come and go.

Choosing to resist a fantasy could also make it difficult for the mind to relax and reach orgasm. You could also affect your arousal if the mind is deprived of sexual imagery. Unusual fantasies are harmless when not acted upon. Paraphilia[22] is the expression used to describe an individual who has to think about one particular fantasy each time to reach arousal, or even climax. This type of fantasy may grow out of control, particularly in relationships.

Rather than focus on your ideal fantasy, allow your mind to create other erotic scenes. I like to meditate, which clears the mind and allows sexual imagery to slip in easily. The image of waterfalls is erotic, playful, and sexy, especially during a hot fantasy. However, if you add the feeling of water or oil on the skin during foreplay, the new sensation will heighten every second of pleasure.

Tie up your partner and dominate him/her with a little role-play to heighten the element of fun in your relationship. Your mind's potency will unleash when you share imagery and discuss these fantasies/fetishes with your partner.

GROUP SEX

Group sex is a usual fantasy for most men. If the aim is to bring this fantasy to fruition, discuss it with your partner beforehand. Do you share a strong connection to your partner after experimentation with swinging, group sex, and orgies? If so, your relationship is very likely to survive further tentative phases. This is important.

A real fantasy that involves domination and/or group sex requires trust between both partners before a final decision is made. Trust your heart, which always speaks the truth. NEVER take part in a fantasy to please a partner, as future problems could occur. You do not want your partner to take advantage and disrespect you by asking you to participate in further real life fantasies. Would it not be better to gain his/her respect by stating a firm no?

Discuss all thoughts, feelings, and negativities with your partner, if they arise. Find out why you both share the desire to explore group sex. Is it a test of trust or do you crave further excitement in your sex life? Some individuals have a natural tendency toward experimental sex. Do not feel guilty if this is you. Instead, choose a partner who reciprocates your desires. If your sex life moved to a kinkier level, would group sex still be a high priority on your sexual agenda?

I once disrespected myself when I told my ex-boyfriend, Jason that I would like to try a threesome with another woman. During the insecure stages of my early twenties, I would have done anything to keep us together. I was far too attached to him, and he affected me emotionally. Consciously, I hated the idea of going against my gut feeling, and I am positive that he lost respect for me that night because our relationship ended soon after. The moral of this story is if you want to experiment with group sex, go for it, but do it only for yourself.

Men, Women, or Both: After a discussion with your partner and you decide that, yes, group sex is the next big move you wish to experience, you must then decide on the gender of the third person. Men are more liable to choose a female, and women will opt for another man, but it is paramount to reach an amicable decision.

If his choice is to invite another female, this may prove difficult for a woman, especially if she is not already bisexual. Men fantasize about lesbian threesomes for the visual image of two women touching and kissing each other intimately. It is natural for a woman to desire two men in a threesome fantasy. Men who already feel comfortable in their own sexuality should have no problem getting naked beside another man, but some men may show homophobic inclinations. This is a form of insecurity, but questioning the motive can successfully defeat it.

During group sex, your partner is still the most important person in the scene. If a man were lucky enough to have two women in his sight during group sex, it would be foolish to expect his partner to participate in a lesbian romp, especially if she does not feel at ease. As a man, put yourself in her place. Would you suck a penis or French kiss a man? If the latter two thoughts turned your stomach, do not expect her to play the same game.

Before the act of group sex, set some rules, e.g. no kissing the "third person" on the mouth. Kissing is a very intimate act for many couples, and to pass the line of trust for borderline entertainment could wreck your strong relationship. Of course, have fun with the rules, but agree that group sex will not alter your future relationship. Will you both be able to move on and forget it ever happened, or will it become a hot fantasy to reminisce of with your partner?

Friends or Strangers: If you or your partner feels attracted to a friend and would like to invite him/her into the threesome fantasy, you must discuss this issue with your partner? Ask yourself if it is a good idea. Can you spot a definite spark between your partner and friend?

Invite your friend for dinner and find out if s/he feels only lust toward your partner. Anything deeper than lust is dangerous territory in which to take your group sex fantasy. Do not put your relationship in jeopardy EVER. However, if you have faith in your heart that no secret rendezvous will take place in the future between your partner and friend, group sex could develop real chemistry between you both. It may be a planned secret that remains between only the three of you— a fun experience to remember when you are all old and wise.

What happens if you decide on a threesome fantasy, but you have no idea of who to invite? Why not place an advert in your local paper for an individual who fits the bill for a no-strings threesome. It may be a healthier option to choose a stranger, rather than a close friend. Beforehand, it is beneficial to meet him/her in a coffee shop or similar venue to ask questions about his/her sexuality. Write a list of questions e.g. have you used condoms with strangers in the past, and when was the last time you had a test for Sexually Transmitted Diseases (STDs) and HIV? Based on his/her answers, make a decision on what your heart states.

After your group sex experience, a stranger is out of touch, but close friends linger. Holding a grudge over a friend is never a positive experience, and this often occurs after an argument or dispute with a loved one or friends. Whoever you decide upon as the lucky "threesome," keep a selection of condoms handy.

Orgies or Swinging Parties: Both of these sexual acts sound similar, would you agree? Couples who attend venues or parties with the specific aim to get passionate with another couple are known as swingers. Alternatively, couples who practice an open-relationship may feel inclined to attend a swinging party.

An orgy often involves having sex with one or more individuals at the same time. If you view a threesome as a "one-off" sexual encounter, then swinging is a regular act between highly sexed couples.

Individuals with an open mind may choose to attend regular orgies or swinging parties. However, these parties are not for the faint hearted. Swinging requires trust and honesty between partners. I admire couples who employ danger into his/her sex life by sharing a partner with another.

For swinging/orgies to work effectively, you must be very comfortable with your sexuality. Do you discuss your innermost thoughts and emotions regularly? Swingers are open-minded and know exactly how to fulfill his/her sexual desires. Private swinging parties provide an evening of spontaneous fun.

If you have jealous inclinations toward your partner, it is perhaps not a wise step to experiment with threesomes, orgies, or swinging, as jealousy can easily make or break a relationship during these precarious sexual acts. Complete trust, honesty, and love are necessary in order for your relationship to survive. After the passionate deed, a strong bond will always bring a couple back together. If the relationship is not based on trust, either of you could easily indulge in a secret affair. Orgies or swinging parties require respect, desire, and admiration for your partner, plus an open mind which allows you to share your private fantasies with other couples.

Some couples become a member of a swinging club, attend orgies, or attend both. There is nothing seedy about these parties, especially if you share an open-relationship or enjoy watching your partner getting intimate with another individual and/or couple. Always use protection throughout your sexual encounters, especially if you decide upon this phase of experimentation. Sharing this level of intimacy with a partner can build a stronger bond, intense orgasms, and unleash your innermost desires.

Other Sexual Acts: Dogging[23] is an act where individuals or couples meet in selective areas, e.g. car parks, woodland areas etc. predominantly to watch and participate in sexual acts. However, you must practice dogging in a safe place away from Government officials, as it could possibly lead to an arrest.

Voyeurism is a similar act where open-minded individuals grow aroused when watching individuals or couples participate in sexual acts, e.g. intercourse and masturbation. There are a huge number of websites that promote voyeurism, and it is far safer to watch from your own home than go on the lookout to get the same kicks. While some websites do request payment, others give you free access to hundreds or thousands of voyeurism movies or live web cams. A lot of kinky individuals grow aroused when another man/woman is watching the intimate act, plus an intimate channel satisfies both parties.

Another very popular sexual act is cottaging[24]. However, if a couple involved in a sexual act are caught by Police officers, especially if they are discovered in a public area, it could lead to a lawful arrest. The public toilet is a very popular area for homosexual men to seek sexual gratification with others.

THE BIG O

ORGASMS

Orgasms are one of the only free and infinite experiences in life—together with sex, love, rain, and air. Individuals who love to experiment with masturbation may be hooked on the wonderful euphoric feelings of contentment before and during climax. I often tell my friends (who use marijuana), have an orgasm instead to achieve a natural high through the release of endorphins.

In women, the vaginal muscles tense during the first stages of arousal, and lubrication is secreted thirty seconds later. As the genitals become excited, the clitoris fills with blood, altering its normal shade of red to a deeper ruby/purple. The nipples and breasts swell in size to match arousal, and respiration and heart rate increases. Women may feel a warm flushing effect against their skin. The vagina lubricates and widens to allow for penetration, and a clitoral orgasm releases a wonderful cascade of muscular contractions in the uterus and outer vagina—the orgasmic platform—before warmth and emotion dominates the body.

Men enter a similar more visible stage. During arousal, the muscles tense and the penis fills with blood creating an erection. The second stage of arousal creates a stronger hardness, and the orgasmic release becomes difficult to control. Ejaculation takes place only seconds after the muscular contractions wave over him during an orgasm. Ejaculation and orgasm differ in men. Some men are able to hold back the ejaculation and enter a multi-orgasmic phase. Masturbation can teach a man self-control. After ejaculation, the orgasm overwhelms the body forcing out short spasms of pleasure, and the penis turns flaccid. Men often require a short period before intercourse or masturbation to allow their testicles to refill with semen.

During orgasm, the sphincter muscles in the anus contract in both men/women. This feels highly pleasurable for a man as the g-spot is situated in this area. However, it may feel slightly weird for a woman. Some orgasms are more powerful than others, which is the primary reason why intense orgasms can affect other organs.

Vasocongestion is the build up of blood that forces the female labia and the male penis to swell. In women, the uterus swells and doubles in size during sexual arousal. After just ten to twenty minutes, the uterus then returns to its normal size.

The limbic cortex is the pleasurable part of the brain, and also causes the insane spurt of electrical energy that is felt directly before orgasm.[25] This section of the brain also controls awareness, and some orgasms can last longer or feel more intense than others during different stages of arousal.

Some individuals would describe an orgasm as simple tension release, while others view an orgasm as seventh heaven. I would encourage everyone to experience a real orgasm through masturbation or sex. It is one of the most potent emotional releases in existence today.

Men and Orgasm: Men are able to experience a multitude of orgasms. It often occurs during lovemaking and masturbation, although some highly stimulated men can reach orgasm without touch, e.g. by performing oral sex on a partner, sharing passionate kisses, reading erotic fiction, or through stimulation of the g-spot situated in the anus.

By practicing self-controlled masturbation techniques, men can reach multi-orgasmic levels of pleasure. However, this is also dependent on a partner, especially if s/he turns you insatiably horny during a sexual encounter.

Women and Orgasm:[26] Clitoral and vaginal pleasure are two of the most popular orgasms to experience amongst women. How this occurs differentiates between women, but some lucky females can orgasm through kissing, fantasy, deep penetrative sex, or even anal sex. During the peak of arousal, women become highly orgasmic. What one woman chooses to experience as pleasure during foreplay or sex, another may choose to ignore. However, the body undergoes intense changes before, during, and after orgasm.

Throughout the menstrual cycle, the sex drive of a woman reaches incredible heights. Although the sight of blood is unpleasant to see, a woman may display a wilder side than she would normally. My orgasms are overwhelmingly powerful during the menstrual cycle. Many women will experience this too. An orgasm also relieves breast and groin pain without painkillers.

Faking Orgasm: If you have never before experienced a real orgasm during sex or masturbation, it is always easier to keep up the pretence by faking orgasm. However, this teaches a partner nothing about your pleasure. Have you forgotten about your sexual satisfaction? You deserve the same pleasure you cause in a partner. Faking orgasm is substandard, and could lead to future relationship problems.

Sex helps to build intimacy between couples, and the majority of couples make love to reach some level of ecstasy. This may be an orgasmic release, to cause your partner's orgasm, or to experiment with kinky foreplay that heightens extrasensory pleasure e.g. domination or asphyxiation.

If your partner does not put in the appropriate time and effort to arouse your sexuality, you need to learn how to tap into the sexual mind and reach orgasm through masturbation or fantasy. Practice this skill until you are able to describe exactly how you love to satisfy your body. Alternatively, confident individuals may prefer to give a partner a private demonstration.

Women enjoy domination as a one-off, but trying to attack her incessantly with a quickie sex session or a deep wet kiss could be a turn off, especially if you are unable to read her body language or be unwilling to put additional time and effort into her satisfaction. However, quickie sex is the perfect make-up sex to have after an argument.

Foreplay can have the same effect on men, especially if a woman treats the penis as a fragile object. Some women like to stroke the penis softly, which is unlikely to create a memorable scene or cause his orgasm. Men prefer to tug the penis harder, especially during masturbation and oral sex.

Both genders vary in how s/he desires touch, especially in the genital region. However, if you are willing to take a leap of faith and confess how you like to be touched, a stronger bond will develop between you both.

Faking Tips To Spot In a Woman

- **The Clitoris**: Is it a dark purple shade and very sensitive to touch after her orgasm? Does she push your hand away from her clitoris directly after her climax? If not, she has probably faked it. After a real orgasm, the clitoris is extremely sensitive to the slightest touch.

- **The Sex Flush**: Do her cheeks flush after orgasm? The flush may also appear on the neck and chest, but disappears equally fast within minutes. See no flush on her body, and she has more than likely faked an orgasm.

- **Vagina**: Women can always fake an orgasm with enthusiastic moans, but during a real orgasm, her vagina contracts sporadically for 3-10 seconds. If you spot no spasms in her vagina, she may have faked her pleasure.

- **Noise**: It is near impossible to stay quiet during a real orgasm. The body shakes, inhibitions disappear, and a satisfied smile dominates her face. I once managed to remain incredibly silent during masturbation in a tent at a festival, while my friend and her boyfriend were asleep. It was an especially horny challenge.

Faking Tips To Spot In a Man

- **Thrusts**: Directly before an orgasm, men thrust harder than they would normally during oral sex or penetration. If he lets you do all the work, even if you are sure he has relieved himself, look for a quivering body, shallow breaths, and deeper thrusts. If you spot neither, he may have faked his orgasm.
- **Noise**: Even shy males get noisy during the real thing. Sex is extremely pleasurable for both parties. If penetration or oral sex does not draw out his fervent moans, how will you know if he has climaxed?
- **Oral Sex**: If you suspect he has faked an orgasm during penetration, perform oral sex on him. It is impossible to notice a faked orgasm during ejaculation. A downside to oral sex could be his inability to relax. This could create performance anxiety and difficulty in reaching heights of ecstasy. I once sucked off a man for over half an hour, but his inability to relax ruined the moment, and he failed to orgasm.
- **Pelvis**: A real orgasm causes his pelvis to contract involuntary. If you do not feel his body move or spasm, he could have faked an orgasm.

Note: Never confess of a faked orgasm. This could cause performance anxiety in your partner during sex and foreplay. Once a lie has been told it is difficult to build trust. Instead, keep quiet and practice solo masturbation to find out which specific thoughts, fantasies, and finger pressures arouse your genitals. Focus on the same throughout lovemaking.

Multiple Orgasms In Men: It is possible for men to reach a multi-orgasmic phase. This rests on how sexually responsive you are to orgasm, and how a partner makes you feel during intimacy. A sensual lover is far more exciting than a sexy woman who remains motionless. Enthusiasm is paramount during lovemaking. If you are a woman who loves to experiment sexually, you will mould into a diamond through his eyes.

After climax, the penis slips into a refractory period where both erection and desire fades. With the right partner, however, the desire to make love should remain. A sleep hormone is released after orgasm, but the drowsiness can be overlooked with horny foreplay.

If your partner is able to make you climax through foreplay, explicit talk, and sexual motivation, you may slip into a multi-orgasmic state. Experiment with the squeeze technique[27] during solo masturbation to lengthen your orgasms.

The Squeeze Technique

1. Get into a comfortable position, take a few breaths to relax, and begin masturbating until near orgasm.
2. When you feel the urge to ejaculate, stop immediately. Squeeze and hold the pelvic floor (PC) muscles—to stop the flow of urination—for ten seconds.
3. Masturbate again and bring yourself closer to ejaculation, before halting the strokes again. Contract your PC muscles and focus on your emotional response and depth of arousal.
4. Take a rest if you must.
5. Stroke your penis again, but allow the waves of orgasm to penetrate your body. Try to notice the spasms that indicate the start of ejaculation inside the pelvis and base of the penis. Throughout orgasm, do not stimulate the penis, but squeeze the pelvic floor muscles tight. There will be a strong desire to ejaculate, but use your willpower to stop the urge.
6. If you ejaculated but want to last longer, continue to practice with your timing.
7. The squeeze technique is manageable with steady practice.

If you can resist the urge to ejaculate during the early stage of lovemaking, a wave of pleasure will energize the body. This is the beginning of multi-orgasmic pleasure. Be patient, but continue to drive yourself to the edge with varied strokes, then allow your orgasm to drift into every pore.

Male Multi-Orgasmic Technique

-   Directly before the release of ejaculation, stop your lovemaking and relax your muscles. At the same time, squeeze the pelvic floor muscles and allow the pleasurable sensations of orgasm to wave through your mind and body.
-   If the penis is sensitive after orgasm, remain in this calm state of tranquility. Initiate lovemaking with your partner when you feel ready for a second explosion. Stop again to reach another multi-orgasmic state.[28]
-   Men can also experience multi-orgasms during ejaculation when the penis experiences partial ejaculations. While a lot of men will lose an erection through this method, other men are able to maintain it and reach mini orgasm after mini orgasm until a final explosion takes hold. It is possible to reach climax, desire it again, and enter a multi-orgasmic state

of bliss. Continue to penetrate your partner, but alert your mind to also focus on your multi-orgasmic pleasure.

Multi-Orgasms in Women: Women can become multi-orgasmic in numerous ways—stimulation of g-spot, kissing, anal sex, and/or clitoral stimulation. The sensitivity of the clitoris starts to wear off minutes after an orgasm, but it is perfectly okay to concentrate your focus on other areas of the body until the sensitivity subsides. G-spot stimulation makes it easy for a woman to experience multi-orgasms during sex.

Clitoral Stimulation

1. During masturbation, rub yourself quickly until you feel on edge to orgasm.
2. Move your fingers to your breasts, and tease the nipples rock hard.
3. Return full focus to the clitoris. The sensation to orgasm will subside, but the mental arousal will remain. Intense excitement and the motivation to orgasm will create spasms in the vagina.
4. Continue to rub yourself quickly then slower to build another orgasmic peak.
5. Keep yourself on edge with gentle strokes—30-60 minutes—to build an orgasm that feels superior.

Female Multi-Orgasmic Technique

- If you have the free time, build yourself into a multi-orgasmic state by visualizing a hot fantasy to stimulate your mind.
- Dip two or three fingers into your vagina to collect the moisture and transfer them to the clitoris.
- Focus your strokes away from the clitoris, which will be growing larger by the second.
- Stroke the outer vaginal lips, but continue to brush your middle finger over the clit.
- Stroke the inner thighs and outer vaginal lips, but resist the urge to rub the clitoris until the impatience to orgasm becomes too hot to handle! This technique builds patience, self-control, intense orgasms, and will turn you wetter than usual.

How To Get Longer Orgasms: Regular masturbation will teach you how to build longer, more intense orgasms. These superior orgasms will feel like you are not only stroking yourself, but your partner is with you too! Work with your partner, or let your mind visualize a hot fantasy that turns you horny in an instant.

If you want to experience intense orgasms, you must first put in the work. Rub yourself to the brink of orgasm, and then stroke your genitals slowly. Continue with this move two or three times until you feel the urge to explode. Regular masturbation makes it easier to train the genitals to contract for longer. I discuss mutual masturbation and how it can build intense orgasms in the "Oral Sex" chapter.

Show Enthusiasm: Help him reach orgasmic ecstasy by displaying an enthusiastic side during oral sex or lovemaking. When men orgasm, it is rarely quiet. His moans, bodily spasms, and the way he urgently grips a favorite part of his partner's anatomy tells a woman everything. Act as if he is the hottest lover in the world.

Meet each of his moans, and ask him to pound you harder. State how good he feels inside you. Ego-boosting comments like this—together with deep reverse thrusts during sex—will push him over the edge. When a man is very sexually forward toward a partner, orgasm will feel strangely different—in a positive way.

During oral sex, make flirtatious eye contact while tantalizing his penis in a variety of ways, e.g. moisturize his tip, lick up and down his twitching shaft, and masturbate him with firm strokes. If your jaw starts to ache, use your fingers, tongue, and lips to push him over the edge. Treat his penis like your favorite sex toy. This will turn him so hot for you that he is likely to experience a strong orgasm, which will also turn the scene memorable.

DESIRE

In order to have mind-blowing sex with your partner, you must both share an equal level of desire. I'm sure you have heard the concept that men think about sex every seven seconds? But many women are also highly sexed. Society makes it hard for a woman to grow in her sexuality, and we are judged if we sleep around, use a man, or disrespect our bodies. If men can do this, why do women not have the same rights? If you get rid of the stigma of peer pressure to conform, and start to love and accept yourself just the way you are, no outside thoughts or judgments will affect you consciously.

I am a highly sexual woman, and through my open sexuality, I found a partner who recommended I write this guide. It has taken me a long time to openly respect my sexuality, as I was brought up to view masturbation and sex before marriage as a sin. Why do I care what people think of me? Judgments are negative, and only an insecure person would judge another. It saddens me that some women will never feel the pleasure of an orgasm as they are forced into circumcision. Most of this is force fed into the subconscious mind through religion or beliefs. How would you feel if your hot spot was gone forever, and you chose to ignore masturbation or wild sex because you had a subconscious belief that it is wrong to experiment? Let's feel compassion for the young women who will never experience this sublime pleasure, and feel gratitude that you have the free will to influence your own mind and genitals if you so wish to. It's time for all women to take back our power and know that there is nothing wrong with solo pleasure.

With the right partner, a woman's sexuality can develop. However, desire must exist between couples. For example, a woman who loves sex four or five times a week, and her partner only twice. Equaled desire will alleviate sexual problems, but lack of desire could cause a partner to look elsewhere.

Desire is the compulsory factor required in a relationship to create fireworks. Foreplay is a great tool, which can be used to build desire. If role-play intrigues you, make a date with your partner and act like you are two strangers meeting for the first time. Does this create the butterfly effect in your tummy, building the same excitement you felt during the early days of your courtship?[29]

All relationships are thrilling during the early days, would you agree? You can't keep your hands off each other, you make love all the time; share long erotic kisses that last from morning to afternoon, and all the senses heighten during foreplay. However, in a long-term relationship or marriage, couples take advantage of each another and expect the same level of desire to remain. All relationships require commitment, dedication, and mutual effort.

Sexual desire demands work, especially over the long-term. Some lucky couples share a great bond, which helps to enhance sexual desire. However, the majority of couples will find that desire starts to wane after just six months. To maintain a strong sexual connection, it is imperative to create an equal level of desire in your partner. Choose to neglect your relationship, and the mixed messages could create a need for your partner to seek an affair. All it takes is one stranger to compliment your partner, which then creates a spark of attraction. If there is an inconsistency of desire in your relationship, future problems could occur.

Romance is a great creator of desire, therefore it is important to spend time communicating, experimenting sexually, and developing the same desire you both shared at the start of your relationship. Low sexual desire is a problem, especially if it is one-sided. This could stem from a lack of sexual initiation, or the failure to respond with arousal when your partner initiates sex. Women are not the only ones who suffer from low sexual desire; men also suffer with this issue. Is it any wonder that most individuals start to panic when desire wanes? Controllable factors could be a prime cause, e.g. medication, depression, smoking, and an unhealthy diet.

Sex is a physical expression of the direction where a relationship is headed. If an individual feels under pressure to perform sexually, lovemaking is unlikely to feel special. Do not have sex to please a partner. There are ways to create desire if it has diminished from your relationship.

Affairs are weak and an easy way to release sexual frustration. In the early days of a relationship, the components of chemistry, personality, attraction, or all three interlock. During the first stage of attraction, flirtation begins. This is important for a woman as it helps her to feel sexy. From a man's perspective, flirtation creates the confidence to take the relationship further.

During the early days of courtship, couples share erotic kisses and experience amazing lovemaking, which makes it difficult to concentrate on much else. Why must those feelings change? Excuses and no effort are only for the weak-willed?

Ask yourself this question. When you met your partner for the first time, what part of him/her did you find attractive? Was it a beautiful smile, a pair of sparkling eyes, or a personality that radiates happiness? Both men/women adore compliments and it takes a confident individual to praise another.

If you have achieved success in a relationship it is obviously for a reason. Whether you have been together for three months, ten years, or fifty years, always find the time to compliment your partner. If you continue to create desire in your partner with kind words and compliments, why would s/he crave desire elsewhere?

Why Does Desire Diminish? Repressed sexual desire could occur for a variety of reasons—low self worth, medication, or stress etc. Most individuals will not own up and state the obvious; s/he would rather have an affair than deal with the underlying problem. Communication is vital when sexual desire falters. Three diverse forces come into play with desire: sexual motivation; sexual desire; and the sexual wish.

- **Sexual Motivation**: A complex and very important aspect of desire is the motivation. Some couples retain the motivation to have sex with a partner through love and respect for him/her. The carnal desire for sex takes over and s/he cannot think of life without sexual gratification. The motivation to have sex is buried deep within the subconscious mind and memories of horny sexual encounters trigger the desire for sex.
- **Sexual Drive**: The drive is the carnal sexual appetite. The hormone responsible for sex drive in both men/women is testosterone, although it is higher in some individuals than others. Sexual drive is important, though motivation may take prime importance over the sexual drive.
- **Sexual Wish**: The wish is the social aspect of lovemaking and the reason why many couples retain sexual intimacy long after his/her biological drive reduces. Sex creates a feeling of excitement, desire, and enthusiasm, which has no direct contact with an individual's sexual appetite.

Example: A woman who craves sex regularly (sexual wish), masturbates often because she needs fulfillment (sexual drive), yet struggles to crave her partner sexually (sexual motive). These varied desires could create problems for some couples.[30]

Creative Ideas To Build Desire

- **Dominate**: Tie up your partner and tease him/her with a feather, ice cube, or piece of silky material until s/he begs for sexual gratification. Drive your partner into a whirlwind of ecstasy.

- **Role-Play**: Agree a role-play fantasy beforehand, and pretend that you have never before met your partner. Examples may include the cinema, bar, library, or supermarket etc. Act completely out of character and have some fun. Build desire by staring into his/her eyes throughout conversation. Wear something revealing and wait for the admiring glances from your partner. Experimenting with role-play gives you the chance to display a side of your character, which your partner may not have noticed.

- **Romance**: If this is not at the top of your agenda, surprise your partner with elements of romance. Buy a single red rose and cook a romantic meal for him/her. Dim the lights, add scented candles to the scene, dress sexy, feed each other, and flirt with your partner.

- **Relieve Tension**: If you often fail to initiate sex, now is the time to show off a dominant side. Down a couple of vodka shots for courage, and when he least expects the attention, pounce on him. Experiment with masturbation to rid the body of sexual tension, especially if you have a varied sex drive to your partner.

- **Flirt**: Compliment your partner every day. The way you make a partner feel is the base definition for a great relationship. The menstrual cycle can affect a woman hormonally; so if she ever displays a moody side, remind her of the positive aspects of her personality that you love.

- **Time**: Communicate with your partner to find out his/her sexual needs. How does your partner like to be touched and kissed? Is your partner timid or experimental? With the appropriate time and effort put forth, your relationship will build in strength.

- **Communicate**: How you communicate to a partner can help you better understand him/her. Trust develops through communication. If you seek the underlying cause of his/her repressed desire and work through those tough times by offering love and support, your bond will strengthen.

- **Touch**: Individuals who lack sexual desire may not realize that touch is absent from the relationship. Touch is a natural human instinct, which everyone craves. Holding hands is important to many couples. However, the most basics of touch, e.g. kissing, hugs, and hand holding often disappear within a long-term relationship or marriage. Paying attention to your partner's feedback during foreplay helps him/her to feel important and re-establishes sexual desire. Add appropriate effort by displaying a romantic side, and your "sparkle" could return.

- **Visit The Doctor**: It could be time to visit your physician, especially if you feel that your repressed desire stems from a hormonal imbalance. Testosterone can be taken in tablet form, although it may require several weeks to take effect.
- **Therapy**: If none of the above tips work and you are fearful of repressed desire affecting your relationship, therapy may be your next option. A specialist expert will communicate with you over several sessions with the aim to discover the underlying cause.

SENSUALITY

KISSING

Kissing is a well-known hot method of seduction. The lips contain rich nerve endings, which work to arouse other hot erogenous zones in the body. A kiss can be sizzling hot and arouse the genitals, but a bad kiss can have the opposite effect. Good kissing technique develops with practice, but it is always better to work with your partner to develop a unique sensual kiss of your own.

During an erotic kiss, the genitals receive a spark of arousal, which then creates a fulfillment to orgasm. Is it not surprising that both the genitals and lips come into contact during a sexual encounter? Both are extremely rich in nerve endings.

Has anyone ever complimented your kissing technique? If yes, this is positive, encouraging, and a great compliment to remember whenever life gets you down. Each individual is unique in how s/he passionately kisses a partner. Remember the "rule" of "adjust to your audience." If your partner's kiss is soft, teasing, and pleasing to your genitals, now is the time to prove you both share great chemistry by simulating his/her smooch.

One glance at a passionate embrace could provoke envy in jaded couples who judge other happy couples. However, with the addition of time, effort and romance, a shaky relationship can strengthen in all areas.

In some countries, kissing is forbidden in public. In the future, if you plan to visit a strict law abiding foreign country like Pakistan or India, you must adhere to their laws. Lack of ignorance could lead to an arrest.[31]

Do Bad Kissers Exist? Most definitely yes, and I have experienced a few during my teenage years. Bad kissers do not have the patience to work with a partner during the moment. It feels unpleasant and does nothing to excite the genitals. In women, it may create the opposite effect—vaginal dryness.

I experienced a horrendous kiss on my seventeenth birthday, which made me gag repeatedly. When I saw the same guy many years later, he was now a taxi driver. I'm not sure why I got in the car, but after he dropped me at home he attacked my mouth again with the same nauseating long tongue before I had to push him away. I dread to think what a kiss under the mistletoe would involve—

sucking my lips until they turned blue perhaps? A bad kisser is also the sign of a selfish partner who does not wish to build up the levels of desire in his/her partner. In my view, a good kisser equals smokin' sex.

A good kiss is achievable by anyone. Kissing requires the skill of instinct and is often performed with the eyelids closed. Lips are full of rich nerve endings, and for many individuals; a hot kiss often feels better than sex. If you *do* close your eyes during a kiss, the sight is excluded, which then heightens the other four senses of touch, taste, scent, and sound. A great kiss is full of synchronicity. Couples work collectively to brush the lips together, melting the tongues in sync to turn a kiss unique.

My first kiss (aged fourteen) happened on the side street with an older man. After a brief flirtation, he asked to kiss me. When it happened, my first thought was, "What if he thinks I'm a crap kisser." He stopped minutes later to compliment my kiss, which overinflated my ego.

If you want to experience a hot kiss that arouses both your physical body and mind, work with your partner to develop sensual kissing games, e.g. suck the top lip gently before teasing the lower lip. Use your tongue with every embrace to turn the scene horny. Do not overlook the power of a passionate kiss. Intimacy is essential to a relationship, but it is especially significant to a woman.

How To Enliven A Boring Kiss: A peck on the cheek does nothing to arouse the genitals. However, if you turn your attention to the neck or earlobes, a simple kiss can create substantial arousal in your partner. A kiss can provoke anyone to crave sexual pleasure, especially if you are confident of which erogenous zones to stimulate on your partner.

Using the tongue during a kiss enlivens the senses of both you and your partner, but experimenting with varied kissing styles also creates desire and ecstasy. Sharing saliva boosts the immune system, reduces the growth of plaque on the teeth, and turns any scene erotic. I once kissed a man who refused to use his tongue. I probed his mouth gently with my tongue, but he wouldn't take the hint.

The Mouth: Licking, tasting, talking, titillating erogenous zones, kissing and smiling all use the key traits of the mouth. Do you use your powerful mouth to its advantage? A simple lick of the lips is a flirtatious move to seduce a man from afar, forcing his thoughts onto your lips.

During a stare from a potential love interest, if she licks her lips slowly she would love to get intimate with you. There is a difference between applying moisture to the lips because of dryness, and seducing a partner with a very seductive lick of the lips. Applying balm, gloss, or lipstick is also a bold move to hook a man, especially if he's already mesmerized by your presence. However, a lot of men struggle to read the body language of women, so if you see this move, take note. *If she licks her lips or applies gloss/lipstick while gazing intently at you, she wants to jump your bones.*

The Wonder of The Lips: The lips are truly magical in how they can arouse any part of the body. Test their sensitivity at any time of the day by closing the eyes and tracing them with a finger. Alternatively, brush your lips over your hand to test the power of the rich nerve endings contained within. Do you feel the sensations fire down to your genitals?

During foreplay, allow your partner to tease your erogenous zones with his lips, tongue, and fingers. A long passionate kiss stimulates the genitals. Focus on the wonderful sensations in the moment to reach a powerful orgasm.

Missionary Position: Many couples enjoy sex in the missionary position because of the ease it allows in kissing a partner. Transferring your lips to another part of his/her anatomy is a confident move. One example is doggy style, e.g. licking up and down the spine, nibbling the earlobes, or kissing the nape of the neck.

The potency contained in the lips gives you the edge to stimulate the entirety of your partner's body. Take advantage of his/her anatomy and experiment with varied positions and sensations.

The Benefits of Kissing: Sharing saliva during a kiss boosts the immune system and reduces tooth decay. During a passionate smooch, the heart rate increases and a surge of adrenaline drifts through the, which boosts the metabolic rate and offers a fantastic calorie-burning workout. A long passionate kiss releases endorphins and natural pheromones. If the kiss feels good and you feel a sexual bond with your partner, you share a connection of true chemistry. Pheromones are silent messengers, which play cupid to create fireworks with a sexually compatible partner.

Kissing also relaxes the muscles of the face and prevents saggy jowls. Would you agree that it is impossible to kiss during a frown? Many individuals close the eyes during a kiss, especially when shallow breaths take over, instantly heightening the sensation and transcending those emotions to every cell of the body. The body and mind willingly gives into the amazing ecstasy, relaxes, and expects more pleasure.[32]

BODY LANGUAGE

Over ninety percent of the messages we sent out to another are subconscious through body language.[33] I like to study people, especially potential love interests on dates. For instance, I like a confident man who loves his own company, drinks socially, does not smoke or fidget with his fingers, wears trendy clothes, and smiles at others without judgment. Maybe I'm asking for too much, but I'm happy to wait until the Universe aligns our meet.

When seeking a partner for a long-term partnership or short rendezvous, try to decipher his/her body language. Read the following tips to find out what your subliminal gestures tell another.

- **The Desperate Individual**: If you catch an individual continually glancing the room, s/he may be on the lookout for a potential match. Some people like to frown or judge others through appearance, but this is a huge sign of insecurity, and a derivative from the negative subconscious mind. A friendly person is always approachable and kind toward others, whether s/he seeks a partner or friendship. If you catch a person looking left, right, and center for attention, this is a subconscious sign of desperation, which attracts anxiety and could lead to an unlikely encounter with a similar likeminded individual.
- **Seek a Confident Man**: A satisfied man does not fiddle with his fingers or bite his nails; he often places his hands in the pocket. Confident men show a side that states, "I am happy as I am," which creates magnetic attraction. A confident man knows exactly what he wants in and out of a relationship; therefore his actions are natural.
- **Nervous People**: These individuals are easy to spot—chewing on nails, glancing at the floor, and unable to make eye contact with others. If your crush cannot maintain eye contact with you, s/he may be nervous or shy. This could act as a repellant toward confident souls.
- **Mirroring**: Does your crush lean toward you during conversation? If yes, this is a great display of attraction. Although this move is subtle, if s/he is stood away from you or glancing the other way, there may be no

romantic interest headed your way. If your love interest mimics your gestures, e.g. when your hand rests on the chin, does he copy your move? Mirroring is a positive sign of sexual attraction. Leg crossing toward a man is also an extremely flirtatious move. There are many subconscious signals of attraction that you may be able to decipher if you remain aware.

- **Playfulness**: Both parties can display a fun cheeky side to a potential love interest. If he brushes a little "invisible" dust off your shoulder or places his hand on the small of your back, he respects you, finds you attractive, and wants to get to know you intimately.

- **Dilated Pupils**: Unless you socialize with drug users, dilated pupils signal attraction toward another. Those with enlarged pupils look more attractive than others who have lentil sized pupils. However, it is difficult to know if your pupils are larger than usual. If your mind is stating, "God, he/she is so sexy," your pupils are going to increase in size.

- **Genuine Smile**: I'm sure you have spotted a fake smile; the lines around the eyes do not crease, and the face is asymmetrical. A natural smile creates symmetry, and the lines around the eyes crease slightly. In fact, it is instinctive to know a real smile from a faked one.

- **The Two Second Glance**: Does your love interest stare at you for two seconds or longer? This is a bold move and indicates sexual attraction. However, a stare longer than two seconds indicates rudeness. If you allow another person to affect your energy, s/he is already within your personal space (energetic field). Turn your back and take a deep breath if you feel an offensive stare from another. Although some individuals like to stare adoringly at a partner, you must first persist to the relationship stage before you realize the romantic stares are an indication of true love.

- **Lick The Lips**: A bold move from a woman is to lick her lips while gazing at her potential prey. Women have the power to draw attention to the body through clothing, make-up, and sexuality. However, drinking through a straw, dotting gloss on the lips, and smiling all draws attention to a pair of shapely lips. Men love the sight of a female pout; its shape, size, and color displays much information.

- **The Triangle**: During a conversation with a man, if he first glances at your eyes, your lips, then over your body, he finds you sexually attractive.

- **Nervousness:** Nervous tension can manifest through shyness by standing or sitting next to a confident individual, or some individuals can affect another person's energy field, creating instant tension. However, if you make eye contact with your love interest, it could be a sign that you find him/her attractive. It is easier to relax and focus during conversation, but when the attentive stares begin, nervous tension can manifest. Let your instinct guide you.

- **Preening and Stance**: Does he stand with his feet facing toward you during conversation? If yes, this is a demonstration of his undivided attention toward you. If he preens himself while you talk, he is trying to get you to notice his masculinity.

- **Twirl The Hair**: Women like to draw attention to the neck; an area that men love to kiss. This move is often subconscious and a flirty move to draw attention to the neck area. If you feel confident, draw your finger around your lips, down your chin, and in between your breasts. This will keep his eyes firmly fixed on you.

- **Display Confidence**: Attractiveness often signifies good looks, but a magnetic personality will draw people to your side. Self-confidence cannot be bought in a jar. Head out on your own instead of socializing in a busy crowd with friends. Have a dance, talk to strangers, and be friendly to everyone you meet. Soon enough, you will be the one who everyone wants to meet. For once, forget about socializing to find a partner and seek fun instead.

- **Let Love Find You**: Have you ever heard the expression, "When you are patient love will find you?" This statement contains truth. To attract a well-matched partner, you must first develop a relationship with the self and love yourself unconditionally. Forgive yourself for every relationship choice, whether good or bad. Be good to yourself. Buy well fitting clothes, eat well, and quieten the busy mind with meditation. After a while, the love that was originally at the top of your agenda will become less of a priority, and you may well meet your next partner in an unexpected way.

EROGENOUS ZONES

A-Z HOT SPOTS

Erogenous zones are the hot spots found all over the body, which arouse the genitals when stimulated. Every individual has one or two favorite hot spots that create fire in the genitals when excited. For women, the nipples, breasts, clitoris, neck, and lips are highly pleasurable areas to arouse. The armpits, testicles, anus, and penis are sensitive areas to excite in men. The ears, buttocks, and scalp are other hot spots to excite in both men/women.

During stimulation to these hot spots, the mind sends a direct signal to the genitals to awaken. The skin is the largest organ in the body and highly sensitive to stimulation. I list an A-Z of horny erogenous zones to excite on your partner's body. Learn them and use each one to your advantage.

Warning: Many of these erogenous zones may not have sparked your sexual interest as areas to stimulate, but they will heighten the arousal in your partner.

- **Anus**: This area is extremely rich in nerve endings. Rim the anus with your tongue, or use toys and fingers to create excitement. It is a highly sensitive area in men because the g-spot is situated approximately two inches inside the anus. If you choose to experiment with anal sex, always use condoms and lots of lubrication as the area could tear easily. Try anal play in the shower when the area is pristinely clean. Another hot erogenous zone to stimulate on men are the **armpits**.
- **Buttocks**: The skin of the buttocks is sensitive to touch, especially throughout massage and finger strokes. Lie face down and allow your partner to stroke the skin of your buttocks with his/her hands or a piece of silky material. The **breasts** and the **back** are other hot spots to excite.
- **Clitoris**: Endowed with rich nerve endings, the clitoris changes to a deep red/purple shade when aroused. Fondle the clitoris during foreplay with a penis, sex toys, or the tongue. Another stimulating area to excite with the tongue is the **chin**.

- **Dick**: Deep moans, visual images, hot fantasies, touch, erotic fiction, and long passionate kisses arouse the dick. Give your partner a long blowjob to remember and keep it slippery with saliva, oil, or food to leave a memorable scene in his subconscious.

- **Ears**: Soft kisses, sucks, or finger massage around the earlobes will drive your partner into a sexual frenzy. One ear may feel more sensitive than the other. Other hot erogenous zones are the **elbows** and **eyelids**.

- **Fingers**: An area that most individuals take for granted are the fingers. Close the eyes to heighten the senses during foreplay. Blindfold your partner, and then tease one or two fingers around his/her lips before exploring the mouth. When he/she sucks your fingers, your genitals will tingle with excitement. Another hot erogenous zone are the **feet**, although most individuals are ticklish.

- **G-Spot**: This hot spot is found in both men/women. It is situated two inches inside the upper vaginal wall in women, and two inches inside the anus in men. Use fingers or toys to stimulate the male or female g-spot and enhance the potency of orgasm.

- **Hands**: Use the hands to perform massage, or stroke your partner's anatomy to excite his/her nerve endings. Twirling the **hair** or gentle hair pulling is very calming during foreplay.

- **Inner Thigh**: Stimulate this highly sensitive area with the fingers, tongue, lips, toys, silky material, oils, food, and/or ice cubes.

- **Jugular Vein**:[34] This area contains two large veins—internal and external—situated in the neck area, which correspond well to butterfly kisses, gentle caressing, and/or sucking. Brushing the lips over her throat may cause her juices to flow, but it is also likely to cause an erection in men.

- **Knees**: An especially hot erogenous zone to lick, stroke, or kiss is the back of the knees. A fondle can be innocent or invoke the senses deliciously, turning any scene erotic. A **kiss** can provoke any erogenous zone to spark arousal in the genital region. Brush your lips slowly over your partner's mouth without using the tongue, and then excite his/her nerve endings by experimenting with hot kisses.

- **Lower Back**: Use your fingers or an ice cube to excite the lower coccyx (tailbone). When stimulated, the lower back can easily stimulate the genitals in both men/women. The **legs** are another hot favorite to massage, lick, and stroke.

- **Mind**: Without the power of the mind, it would be impossible for the genitals to reach arousal. Stimulate the mind with thoughts of kinky fantasies, or use explicit words to excite your partner. Play out your exact fantasy while rubbing yourself to a powerful orgasm.

- **Nose**: The tip of the nose is a hot spot to kiss in men. Alternatively, blindfold your partner to excite the senses before stroking his nose with a piece of silky material. Other hot erogenous zones are the **nipples** and the **neck**.

- **Odor**: Pheromones are found naturally in body odor. Are you drawn to the nape of the neck, chest, armpits, testicles, or vagina? Let your partner's scent guide you to his/her favorite hot spots.

- **Perineum**: The area between the testicles and the anus, which requires only slight stimulation to turn the penis rock hard. In some men, it could provoke an orgasm or pre-ejaculation to seep out of the tip. The pain of a toy or finger stimulating the anus—male g-spot—is quite a turn on for experimental men.

- **Quadratus Lumborum**:[35] This versatile muscle has many uses, e.g. it performs a side bend, raises the hips, and stabilizes the lower back. Use the lips, tongue, fingers, toys, food, or piece of material to kiss fondle, or stroke this hip area.

- **Radius**: The longest bone in the forearm, which feels sensitive to touch when stimulated with a fingernail or brush of the lips. To further heighten the pleasure, tease over this area with a feather.

- **Spine**: Tickle, kiss, use an ice cube, or brush a feather or silk scarf along your partner's spine. This area contains rich nerve endings and stimulation on this area will cause arousal in your partner. Rub your lips over your partner's spine in the morning to awaken his/her genitals. Any area of the **skin** is another highly sensitive area to fondle and kiss.

- **Tongue**: Also the strongest muscle in the body, the tongue is a fun toy to use which energizes other areas of the body. Another area to fondle in a man is the **testicles**.

- **Urethral Orifice**:[36] This tiny slit in the tip of the penis secretes both urine and semen. Excite this sensitive area with the tongue, lips, fingers, or toys.

- **Vagina**: The female g-spot is situated approximately two inches inside the upper vaginal wall. When aroused, the vagina lubricates and widens to fit the penis during sexual intercourse.

- **Words**: Explicit words stimulate the mind and genitals. Write a story together or read a horny tale to create an erotic scene.
- **Xiphoid Process**:[37] Situated in the sternum—middle of the ribs in the chest area. Stir your partner into a frenzied state by kissing, fondling, rubbing, and caressing this area with your fingers, lips, and tongue.
- **You**: The human body is full of rich nerve endings that heighten during specific foreplay moves, e.g. hot passionate kisses, oral sex, and massage etc. In fact, any careful stimulation on the body with the fingers, tongue, or lips will excite the genitals, especially if you relax and focus on the pleasure.
- **Zonula Ciliaris**:[38] A small muscle that holds the lens of the eye in place. Ask your partner to close his/her eyes before planting soft butterfly kisses over this area, awakening the arousal in his/her genitals.

FOREPLAY FUN

ABOUT FOREPLAY

The thought of foreplay can make a man frown, but fear not girls. It's time to bin the selfish lover who cares only about his pleasure. Some sensitive men love kissing and touching a partner to create her arousal and pleasure. Oral sex, domination, phone sex, kinky toys, and rubbing are just a few of the foreplay methods I discuss in this chapter.

Visual images excite men, but women require direct stimulation. Reading erotica and fantasizing helps to create arousal. Women crave touch, kisses, and stimulation, which build a compatible bond with a partner. Women require time, patience, and foreplay to reach arousal and orgasm. Erotic kissing is a start, but bodily caressing and masturbation require time and effort. Foreplay does not have to be incorporated into every sexual encounter, e.g. quickies or outdoor sex. The former activity stimulates the animalistic side in both men/women, and foreplay can be thrown to one side, as kissing and wild sex is enough. However, foreplay can feel hotter than sex for many couples.

The fun foreplay methods throughout this guide can turn your sex life from boring to sizzling hot. For example, rubbing foreplay creates arousal through the forbidden kiss. Rubbing without kisses heightens the sense of touch and creates a desperate yearn to engage in the most basic of foreplay moves. The rubbing method requires concentration, patience, intense eye contact, and the mental concentration to avoid penetrative sex and smooching.

Continue with foreplay until you both reach a state of sexual ecstasy. Create pleasure in your partner, and s/he will crave you sexually. With the appropriate methods and full concentration given to each, foreplay turns every scene memorable. Foreplay unleashes the sexual energy hidden within your mind, which then awakens your genitals.

A passionate kiss between couples feels exciting when you feel the sexual chemistry running through your body. Begin the multi-orgasmic process by surprising your partner with a wet kiss that releases his/her conserved sexual energy. An innocent neck massage may not create a sexy scene, but when you provoke the scalp with your nails, your genitals will reach arousal.

Foreplay is not boring, especially if you choose to open up the mind and experiment with various methods. Women desire a partner to touch, kiss, and fondle the body. Solo masturbation feels amazing, but only by allowing your partner to caress your clitoris will you learn how to relax the body and reach a heightened state of arousal. Spend time and effort on your partner's pleasure, and his/her arousal will spark the sexual curiosity in your mind to repay him/her with an equal or hotter encounter.

In general, women crave touch and excitement, yet she may not readily confess of her deep "emotional" extras. Tell your partner about your primary sexual needs. If you struggle to orgasm and require more time spent on foreplay, you must be open and honest of this fact. Describing your sexual needs to a partner is nothing to feel ashamed about. If you hanker for attention—ask, or initiate desire by stimulating his/her earlobes with your wonderful tongue.

Women require attention, compliments, and a caring partner to fulfill her sexuality. Give her what she desires and it could unleash her inner minx. Men need only to glimpse the sight of a sexy woman, view a pornographic movie, or read explicit stories to excite the genitals. However, women often require direct stimulation to achieve the same effect.

Both men/women are incredible sexy creatures with diverse needs. While women require time, effort, and foreplay to grow sexually liberated, men should be left alone to view porn, read explicit magazines, or admire a female from afar to emboss his freedom. Neither of these male traits calculates as cheating so learn to trust him. Men and women have very different thought patterns.

Length of Foreplay: This varies greatly between women. A cheeky squeeze of the breasts or a long erotic kiss will create arousal in a partner after twenty short minutes of foreplay. Shy women may require longer methods of foreplay to gain the same level of confidence.

I love foreplay and how it increases the need for sexual gratification. Using foreplay in a loving relationship teaches a man to slow down and focus on self-less pleasure. Men who grow excited by the sight of a naked partner are forced to develop the art of patience. Would you work harder for your own orgasm if you knew you were transmitting ecstatic pleasure to her genitals?

Tease your dick by practicing multiple foreplay methods on your partner, and the whirlwind of passion you create in him/her will creep into your own sexual mind. Not only will your partner build up his/her levels of arousal, but it will also unleash the power of your mind to take charge of his/her pleasure. Foreplay leads a man to crave a partner's sexual fulfillment.

Women love foreplay as it builds up the romantic elements of sex and creates a strong level of intimacy between couples. During the act of cunnilingus,[39] it is easier to reach climax by relaxing the body and mind into synchronicity. Mutual masturbation requires confidence and relaxation during this very intimate act.

Insecurities displayed during the act of foreplay or sex could pose a problem for some couples. Women must learn to push through those uncertainties when they arise. Love yourself unconditionally and do not feel guilty or blame yourself for who you are. View yourself in a positive light, just as your partner sees you. Instead of spotting the flaws, which everyone has—embrace them. Society teaches us to seek outer beauty to create perfection, but this is an illusion. Flaws are not always external. Internal flaws include guilt, insecurities, judgments, hatred, fear, and the inability to forgive others.

Your partner is with you because of the way you make him/her feel. Do not feel guilty or judgmental toward yourself for attracting a great life partner. Moreover, it can be difficult for women to climax during intercourse. You must learn to let go of the outside world and notice the beauty already surrounding you. Practice deep breaths during oral sex and/or mutual masturbation. This is essential if you want to reach orgasm successfully, plus it assists in two ways: (1) you look desirable to your partner, and (2) by climaxing; you boost his ego.

After experiencing the fun elements of foreplay, you may enjoy relentless pleasure with other methods. Holding hands or spending a romantic evening with your partner is satisfactory foreplay for many women.

Flirtatious Suggestions To Try In Public

- **Use Clues**: Design a signal that allows you both to recognize when sex has moved to the top of your agenda. The signal could include a cheeky wink while sucking a finger seductively, or having a secret game of footsy[40] under the restaurant table while you dine out. Take advantage of your partner by displaying sexy clues that indicate, "God, I can't wait to get you into bed."

- **Rubbing**: During intimate foreplay, rub her clitoris gently with your hard penis, or use a finger to penetrate her vaginal wall to mimic the way you love to stroke your dick. Does she enjoy deep finger penetration? If she gives great feedback through hungry moans and a writhing body, superb! Contrary to this move, most women prefer tender strokes, especially during oral sex and masturbation. Women prefer to suck a penis softly, mimicking the way she rubs herself during masturbation. However, this could feel unsatisfactory for men who require a more forceful tug to reach orgasm. Under these circumstances, it is important to communicate your concerns, if any. Homosexual couples are better able to understand a partner's body by identifying how soft or hard to rub the genitals during oral sex. Women understand why breast tenderness occurs throughout the menstrual cycle, and men understand the depths of rubbing and sucking, which are necessary to achieve superior orgasms.[41]

- **Heighten The Senses**: During an evening out with your partner, allow him/her to feed you dessert. This is an incredibly erotic move, especially for couples who have not yet ventured out of his/her comfort zone and chosen to focus on the senses of touch and taste. Close the eyes to heighten the senses further. When the lips, tongue, and genitals are forced to conserve the unique sexual energy within, the mind enters a heightened state of awareness. Avoid touch during romantic foreplay. Feed each other tasty food to test the power of restraint, and heighten your sexual awareness. Continue until the urgent desire for raunchy sex dominates your mind.

- **Sexy Clothes**: Dress sexily for your partner, and allow your flirtatious body language to create fireworks in his boxers, or her panties.

- **Reminisce**: Talk dirty, but avoid touch. Flirty conversation with a partner during a romantic date builds fond memories, pushing your mind into a reminiscent phase of hot first dates, passionate kisses, and glorious full days and evenings spent together in bed.

- **Communicate**: Build up your levels of intimacy and a strong bond through foreplay. Good communication is a useful tool, which builds intimacy in and out of the bedroom. It reminds you that s/he is not only your sexual partner, but your best friend too.

HOT FOREPLAY METHODS

The following three hot foreplay methods have never failed me to turn a man rock hard. Both parties can use these methods to turn his/her partner weak at the knees. The first method—hair massage—could feel like a chore for some men, but the horny effect it will have on his partner is worth the effort. Deepen your moans; feel every second of pleasure, and your levels of sexual desire will grow profoundly.

Hair Massage: A sensational foreplay method I like to use on men after a first date, or when I feel horny and need to initiate sex quickly. Women can use this method to stimulate their partner's scalp and cause genuine pleasures. If you are ever on the receiving end of this fabulous foreplay, I'll be very surprised if it does not relax your body and unlock your mind to horny thoughts.

If you loathe your hair massaged, pulled or played with, move to the next method—the buttock massage. Gentle hair massage relieves stress in the muscles. Both the body and genitals deepen in arousal when the mind relaxes. Use your fingertips to stimulate your partner's scalp, which can be performed anywhere— during a romantic stroll, in a club, swimming pool, or during a romantic meal out together, etc.

1. To use this method to grab the attention of a potential partner, push your fingers slowly into the nape of his/her neck to stimulate the scalp gently. Wait for a reaction. If it is a glorious moan and s/he throws back the head, continue to turn him/her into your little sex toy. If not, massage the nape of the neck, wait for a reaction, and move in with the gentle hair massage. Both men/women will enjoy this sensational foreplay move. Scalp massage or hair pulling releases the tension that can cause migraines or pressure in the shoulders. This move works perfectly to diminish stress. Hair massage turns a non-sexual scene erotic and works magically to awaken the genitals.

2. When the fingernails creep into your partner's scalp, pull on his/her hair gently. If you get a loud groan, experiment with a deeper pull. The prime aim of hair massage is to create arousal quickly. Listen to your partner's reaction, and I guarantee there will be positive feedback of some kind.

3. If you are on the receiving end of hair massage, you must know instinctively that every moan of feedback you deliver is affecting your partner's genitals. Pretty soon, your partner will attack your neck with fervent kisses. Realize that you have used your sexual power to create arousal in him/her.

4. This method of foreplay combines relaxation, pleasure, and erotic thoughts. Use those emotions to your advantage.

Scalp massage or gentle hair pulling can turn any scene erotic. As well as boosting the sex life, one of its prime benefits is to stimulate hair growth. The Orgasmatron[42] is a uniquely shaped tool, which creates endless jolts of pleasure down the spine when used on the scalp.

I have met more than enough men who initially frowned when I requested a hair massage—until my horny side unleashed. This method works a treat on shy men. Hair massage will draw out a horny side in you both, especially if your sole aim is to create his/her pleasure. As soon as you manically writhe against your partner or moan his/her name, all negative doubts subside. I challenge you to find out if hair massage works its magic for you.

My male friend and I got horny one morning with hair massage. While still half asleep, he woke me up by pulling on my hair, knowing this is my only weakness. Although I knew it was wrong as we both had partners, I could not ask him to stop. Of course, I moaned and drooled from both lips the longer he continued. He admitted later that he was rock hard, but we resisted the devilish temptation to take it further.

Heighten The Senses

During scalp massage or hair pulling, blow gently against your partner's neck to send a wave of shivers down his/her spine. Closing the eyes when receiving a hair massage heightens the sense of touch, taste, scent, and sound. Use both the nails and fingertips to stimulate the scalp. Run your nails through a man's scalp and it could cause an erection. Work on all areas of the scalp and practice deeper hair pulls. Remain patient for feedback. Run your fingertips or nails over the nape of his/her neck slowly, before slipping your hands into the scalp.

Buttock Massage: This works very similarly to the hair massage, as it calms the mind and releases tension in the body via touch. Unlike the hair massage, which can be performed anywhere; the buttock massage is best carried out in a relaxed environment. Use a professional massage table if you have one handy.

If your partner is a buttock man, massaging this area will create his arousal. If his hands get a little cheeky throughout the massage, let him stimulate the inside of your thighs. This move relieves stress, opens the sexual mind to fantasize, and turns you both horny.

1. Ask your partner to lie face down on the bed, sofa, or massage table, while naked or fully clothed. Rub your hands over his/her buttocks firmly. If naked, cover your hands in oil, and massage the cheeks firmly. Pummel the buttocks until you hear exhilarating moans flowing off your partner's tongue. Stimulate the inner thigh with a gentle brush of your fingertips. His/her genitals will receive a bolt of ecstasy every time you massage the inner thigh.

2. After fondling the inner thigh, return your hands to the buttocks. Focus on each cheek, and listen carefully for your partner's moans. The gentle caressing of the inner thighs has heightened his/her senses profoundly. This will be noticeable through fervent moans and requests for further satisfaction.

3. If your partner requests a deeper massage, glide your fingers gently over the buttocks to force him/her to beg for pleasure. Gentle strokes create a deeper yearn for further satisfaction.

Note: Do not caress your partner's genitals during the buttock massage. This form of resistance foreplay is designed to pump out all the sexual desires hidden within the mind of your partner.

Heighten The Senses

Strip off your clothes and focus full attention on your partner's buttocks. Soften your touch to drive him/her to crave your touch. Your partner's arousal will magnify yours. This teaches the mind and body to crave exciting foreplay, without a need for sexual gratification. When you both decide that enough is enough, pounce on your partner, rubbing your naked bodies together. This will generate a sexual tension that cannot be ignored.

Advantages of Touch: The hair and buttock massage takes full advantage of the basic survival instinct of touch. They are simple, yet fully effective as they stimulate every nerve ending in the body. When the mind is relaxed, it is better able to surrender to pleasure and enter a multi-orgasmic phase.

The scalp is sensitive to any form of touch, and when stress releases through massage, your partner's desire will build. Why the buttocks you may wonder? Men love all aspects of the female body, but the buttocks are an area where most women feel paranoid. It's time to forget about your flaws, and allow your partner to give your ass the love and attention it deserves. It not only feels great to be on the receiving end of a buttock massage, but it also stimulates each nerve ending in the body.

Rubbing Foreplay: It feels incredible to rub against your partner in clothes, underwear, or completely naked. Rubbing against your partner fully clothed builds patience, self-control, and intense sexual vibes. Although there are three stages to rubbing foreplay, start slowly with fully clothed foreplay before moving onto the advanced stages.

Rubbing foreplay feels erotic. If you have never put forth the time for foreplay in the past, this method will turn on the mind and genitals simultaneously. With the avoidance of specific foreplay moves, e.g. kissing and intercourse, lust and desperation for sexual gratification is created in the mind and body.

Erotic thoughts will dominate the mind, especially if you have the patience to continue with rubbing foreplay for over half an hour. Try this move anywhere that tickles your fancy—sofa, bedroom, cushioned floor, or even outdoors etc. It is perfectly okay to orgasm without sex or sensual kisses, and I hope this method of foreplay turns you both multi-orgasmic.

Stage 1: Rubbing Fully Clothed: During this very early stage of rubbing foreplay, keep the clothes on. By the end of this first stage, you may feel desperate to move onto stage two or three. If you are able to handle this intense first stage, move onto "Heighten The Senses."

- Lie below or on top of your partner fully clothed.
- Grind against him/her. Feel the sensual intensity rise in your mind and genitals. Move your face closer toward your partner, and stare into his/her eyes, willing him/her to break the rules with a kiss.

- Continue to rub your clothed bodies together, building a slow or faster rhythm.

- Soon enough, the lust to strip your partner will rise to the top of your sexual agenda. However, do not give into this ego boost. If you feel close to climax, rub your bodies frantically to release the pleasure, then build up the rhythm again.

- Talk dirty and confess of every thought dominating your mind. Whisper beside his/her ear to stimulate the senses. The ears are a very sensitive erogenous zone to stimulate, e.g. through the heat of a breath, kisses, or sucks. Excite this area and allow the sexual energy to move toward your genitals.

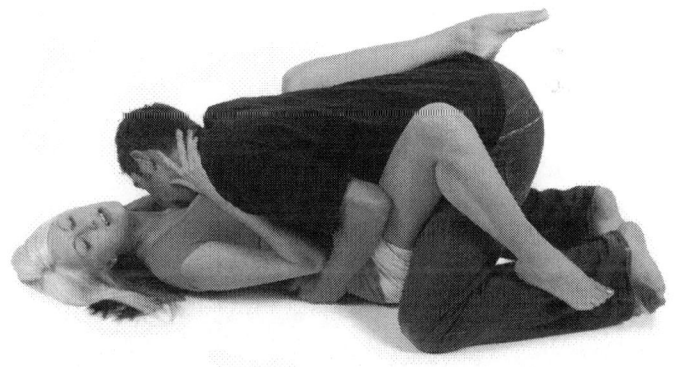

- You may feel an urge to orgasm through penetration or masturbation. Rub together until you reach orgasm, but avoid penetration and kissing on the mouth. Do not let impatience rule your emotions. If you cannot handle the pace, you need to slow down and be aware of your bodies grinding together.

- Continue to bump groins while he brushes his lips against yours, and whisper explicit words beside his ear. You should definitely be feeling more than a little frisky at this stage. Examples of what to whisper could include:

  o "This feel so unbelievably horny."
  o "I want you to bend me over and fuck me hard."
  o "You ready to give in and fuck me nice and hard right now?"

    o   "Do you know how hard/wet you turn me?"

    o   "Bet you are desperate to rub your dick against my bursting clit?"

- Tell your partner how horny you feel. State how much you crave and respect him/her for causing insanity in your sexual mind.
- When neither of you can hold back much longer, strip off your clothes, but cover the genitals. Brush your lips over his/her cheeks, eyelids, nose, and neck, anywhere but the sensuous lips.
- Rub your body against his/hers for up to half an hour without kissing or oral sex. Can you handle the intensity?

Heighten The Senses

Continue the fully clothed rubbing foreplay for up to an hour without sensuous kisses or sex. This early stage of rubbing foreplay will develop the art of patience, but also create an irate level of desire for your partner. Kiss everywhere but the mouth. Brush the lips over the neck to heighten the senses in your partner. Grind your bodies together to achieve a multi-orgasmic state where every brush of his/her lips keeps you on red alert for more. Move to stage two when you wish to take patience a step further.

Stage 2: Rubbing With Underwear: Strip off your partner's clothes, and rub together wearing only underwear.

- Rub your body against your partner's semi-naked body and enjoy the sensations. If you want to add an erotic element, cover your bodies in oil.
- Kiss everywhere on the body, except the mouth and genitals. Talk dirty, create desire with kisses, and rub manically.
- When covered in oil, every sensation feels intensely erotic, which could cause an orgasm in most individuals.
- Whisper your fantasy beside his/her ear, and describe it in graphic detail.
- Heavy breaths and dilated pupils indicate sexual attraction, and this should be evident at this raunchy stage.
- Continue to rub each other while semi-naked for at least thirty minutes. Rub your covered genitals together until you orgasm.

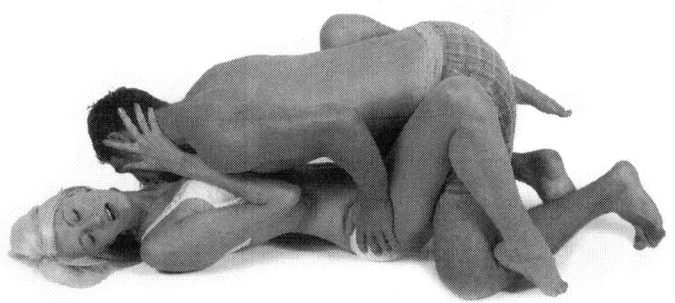

Heighten The Senses

Blindfold your partner throughout this second stage. Limiting one of the five senses automatically heightens the other senses, especially touch and sound. The instinctive way your lips seek out another is a statement to how powerful the senses work in everyone. Kiss everywhere on the body except the mouth and genitals. Nibble the Adam's apple, nose, and eyelids on a man to heighten his senses. The neck, ears, and breasts are hot erogenous zones to titillate in women. Focus on every sensation you experience in the nerve endings. If you can, continue this horny foreplay for up to an hour, and build your bodies into a multi-orgasmic state.

Stage 3: Rubbing Naked: Although this is the toughest stage of all three, there is also the release of penetration and passionate kisses at the finale. The early stage of rubbing naked requires patience and strong self-control. If you crave further excitement, cover yourselves in massage oil, and glide together. An altered sensation felt on the skin immediately heightens the senses.

Usual foreplay allows kissing on the mouth, but focusing your touch elsewhere and adding intense eye contact and explicit conversation is guarantee to drive you both crazy with lust.

- Lie naked beneath or on top of your partner.
- Glide your fingers over his/her body, and purposely rub your genitals together. Refrain from kissing on the mouth or sexual intercourse,

although this will require strong persistence to continue. If you feel flirty and sexual, talk dirty while staring into your partner's hungry eyes.

- Cover your bodies in oil and rub together. Two oily bodies rubbing together will create difficulty in avoiding penetration.

- By this stage, you may have climaxed several times. Thoughts of penetration and hot kisses will be dominating your mind.

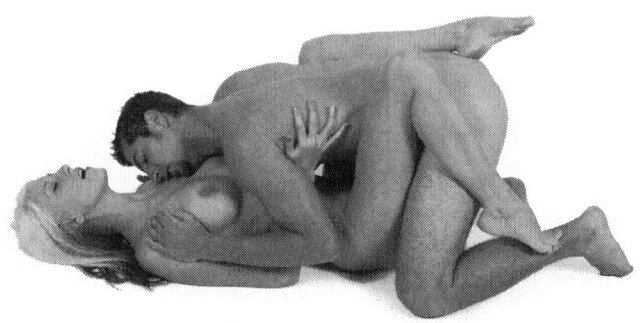

- Time will pass slowly, especially during a horny situation like this. The constant rubbing of a penis over the clitoris can create multi-orgasms in both partners.

Heighten The Senses

Focus full attention on your partner. Forget about the pleasure flowing through your loins, and work on creating pleasure in your partner's hot spots—ears, neck, nipples, and spine. Flip your partner onto his/her front and lick up and down the spine. If you prefer to rub face to face, divert his attention by covering your breasts in oil, and massage his dick in between them. Use a full bottle of edible massage oil and lick each other during your slippery rub. Rub together for up to an hour, or take control of each other with handcuffs and a blindfold. Creating the desire for a kiss and penetrative sex fuels extra potency in your mind. This new energy will swirl through your body and mind continuously until an orgasmic explosion takes hold. Can you handle the heightened sensations for up to an hour without intercourse or passionate kisses?

Continue with the three stages of rubbing foreplay for as long as you can control yourselves. This foreplay builds deep intimacy and powerful orgasms, which feel like a wave of new energy running through your veins—not the usual tension release of a climax.

Hot Foreplay Methods: Other than my three favorite foreplay moves, I believe touch is vital in order to transfer your sex life to intense. Touch is meaningful and expresses thought, love, desire, and affection. Whenever touch fades throughout a relationship, a couple must collaborate and find a way to reinstate that same level of desire. Ask yourself if you still love and desire your partner sexually? Ask appropriate questions to your psyche[43] to try and determine why your sex life is lacking sparkle.

Take advantage of the five wonderful senses—touch, taste, sound, scent, and vision—through awareness and focus during foreplay. The aim of this guide is to enhance every sexual experience through use of the mind—the hottest erogenous zone in the human body.

Add scope and adventure to your sex life by trialing new techniques. If you are used to vanilla sex,[44] why not take a step out of the ordinary and experiment. The following thirteen foreplay methods create fireworks and ensure that neither you nor your partner will fall asleep before, during, or after intercourse.

If you and your partner have sex a couple of times per week and the sexual chemistry is still very much alive, but you need a jolt of passion, this guide will offer you advice and possibilities to enhance your sex life. Does your partner prefer routine sex or a spontaneous encounter? To add fireworks to any relationship, you first need to learn to open your mind to its potential. Although the changes to your thought pattern could be surprising, your mindset will soon focus on passionate encounters. Furthermore, you can ask yourself questions, e.g. "How can I drive my partner crazy with sexual desire." Soon enough, the solution will manifest. The mind is designed to resolve problems.

I have a love of spontaneous sex. The buzz of sexual experimentation intrigues me. Missionary sex is occasionally hot, but I could not cope with it daily. I believe in the power of chemistry, which is why I have discussed natural pheromones in a previous chapter. These natural scents play cupid to help you find a sexually compatible partner better matched to your DNA.

During the early stage of your relationship, did you feel a strong sexual chemistry with your partner? If yes, you can recreate that spark by experimenting with the seductive methods of foreplay in this chapter. Allow your hidden desire to return naturally.

A long term relationship or marriage is special, and must be cherished. Do not take advantage of your partner when love stabilizes. Relationships become comfortable, and the effort required to please a partner sexually could diminish or disappear altogether.

Many couples still believe that the original hot sex will remain if true love exists in the relationship. Truthfully, ALL relationships require hard work and commitment. There are good and bad patches in all relationships. Do not take advantage of your partner or expect that the original "spark" of romance will remain without ample effort.

I respect couples who spend quality time together to communicate, touch, and build up levels of intimacy. Individuals may choose to display this through cuddles, foreplay, communication, romance, and compliments. Successful couples make time for each other in all areas of life. This is vital!

Unfortunately, the daily stresses of life can add great strain to a relationship for many couples. Work is tiring as it zaps energy, which makes it arduous to contemplate sex or foreplay. If work really is that stressful, quit! Money or lack of it creates anxiety, but know that when you are happy and joyful in the moment, you attract great opportunities like a magnet. Do not use work as an excuse to shut down and forget about your relationship.

It is worthwhile to relax with a partner without focusing on sex or foreplay. Stress manifests through joint pain, muscular aches, and aggression. If you sense one of these transformations in your partner, massage his/her neck and shoulders to gently disperse the tension. As touch is often the first sense to vanish when a relationship turns rocky, it is also the one sense that can heal a relationship.

Question Your Relationship

- Look at your partner and note which physical characteristics you love about him/her. Reminisce of great memories and the early days when sex was at the top of your agenda. Listen to your heart and trust your instincts. Do not allow your partner to view your notes.
- Again, try to remember the early days of your courtship. How difficult did you find it to get out of bed?
- Question your mind and investigate why your sex life has become dull or non-existent. What are your instinctive answers? Is the "problem" due to work, lack of desire, infidelity, jealousy, trust, or a stress related problem? Worry is the one emotion that can cloud sane thoughts, but only true

awareness can create credible solutions. Practice meditation or deep breaths whenever you feel tense, or use homeopathic remedies. Have you heard the phrase, "Sleep on it?" When the conscious mind is asleep, your thoughts are resting, but the subconscious mind is still very much awake, trying to absolve solutions to problems. If you feel tension rise because of a relationship problem, hand the problem to your subconscious, and awaken with a clear solution.

- Do you cherish touch and romance in your relationship? Do you share fun dates, which allow you to build on pleasures and sensuality?

- Write down all the ways in which your partner makes you happy. Is there a loving gesture that sends you weak at the knees? Remember why you fell in love with your partner, recall that emotion, and fall in love all over again.

Do you feel more confident about where you stand in your current relationship? In addition, being truthful to yourself draws attention to why you have reached this struggle. Can the situation be altered to positive? Of course, by communicating with your partner, eliminating selfish behaviors, and sharing your life with him/her. A great relationship creates oneness, not separation.

Domination: Does it feel liberating to take control of your partner in the bedroom? Rid the mind of the misconception that domination is rude and only tolerable by professional dominatrices. Buy a good kit that includes a whip, handcuffs, and rubber clothing. Perhaps you have a new style of domination. The world is your oyster! Tie up your partner with handcuffs or a silk scarf, and take charge of him/her in your own distinctive way.

Usual beginner bondage kits from a sex shop often include a whip, blindfold, and handcuffs. Tie up your partner and design a tough question and answer game that you know s/he will struggle to answer. For every wrong answer, your partner is spanked. If the result is in built aggression, whip him/her a little harder. Slight pain given during foreplay enhances the pleasure. Work with your partner to create a unique style of domination.

Heighten The Senses

Domination is not for the faint hearted; it requires confidence in both body and mind. Tie up your partner, and entice him/her with a sexy outfit. Perform a slow strip tease, melt against the wall, and rub yourself to a frantic orgasm.

Alternatively, sit above your partner and massage your breasts, or allow your partner to rub his dick over your genitals while you are tied up and unable to move. If you love the feeling of his/her genitals rubbing you into an amazing frenzy, sit on your partner's face, and give him/her a close up of your aroused genitals. The latter move requires focus, self-confidence, and is not for everyone.

The Edge And Beyond: Blindfold your partner, and tie up his/her hands to create slight discomfort. Sit on top of your partner, and plant an erotic kiss on his/her lips, while brushing your stiff nipples/dick over your partner's chest. If you also decided to blindfold your partner, now is the perfect opportunity to heighten his/her senses during mutual masturbation. With your partner's hands tied, stroke your genitals to a hot orgasm, while s/he watches. Continue to push your partner over the edge.

Take charge by displaying who is the "boss" during this particular game. If you sense frustration building in him/her, or you want to give your partner a quick release, take back your power and remember the art of patience is necessary.

Brush a feather or piece of silky material over your partner's body until the skin turns taut with goose bumps. Experiment with varied ways to dominate your partner and create his/her ecstasy. Whisper a filthy fantasy beside his/her ear. If you spot resistance, punish your partner by rubbing your breasts/dick against his/her mouth. Be creative.

Heighten The Senses

Dominate your partner by sliding your naked body over your partner's while s/he is blindfolded with the hands also secured. Stimulate each erogenous zone with your tongue to create his/her impatience. The key is to only relieve the orgasm when your partner has learnt to control his/her patience and emotion. On release of your partner's climax, s/he will be ready to pounce.

Bondage And Spanking: The film, Secretary[45] exploits bondage and spanking throughout its storyline. Spanking is predominately used by a dominatrix to "treat" her clients. For other individuals, BDSM type activity can turn into a fetish, especially if you have to fantasize about bondage or spanking in order to reach arousal.

However, when used throughout foreplay and fantasy, spanking is a fun element to incorporate into your sex life, which will also enhance the power of your sexual mind. There is nothing seedy about submissive play.

Heighten The Senses

Spanking is one form of BDSM role-play. Old-fashioned couples may deem it kinky, but use your sexual mind to design a game that incorporates gentle spanking when your partner disrespects you. The further mischievous s/he acts, the "harder" the punishment. As the receiver of the spanking foreplay, swear, snarl, or try to fight your way out of the chains or cuffs to infuriate your partner. Spanking incorporates both pleasure and pain. Alternatively, tie up his/her arms and legs, and stimulate the skin all over with gentle whips to turn on every nerve ending in the body. Soon enough, his/her genitals will fire until sexual energy is swirling around every nerve ending in the body, building an incredible orgasm that will only release when YOU decide.

Food Play (Sploshing): Add an erotic element with sploshing. Feed your partner with tasty delights e.g. strawberries, cream, chocolate, or other edible treats. To further stimulate the senses, blindfold your partner, and tease the food in between his/her lips to build satisfaction and desire. When you sense his/her enjoyment, pull away the food and saturate the nipples or genitals. This is fun foreplay at its best and creates an erotic sensation if you choose to develop it further.

Some couples like to fully submerge in liquids and writhe around before having messy sex. If food play appeals to your curious side, spray whipped cream on your partner's body, or rub a strawberry into the skin and lick it off. Play with sweet treats, e.g. fruits, cream, ice cream, cake, rice pudding, and custard.

Alternatively, if you prefer a quick way to create the same sensation, use a full bottle of edible massage oil. Food play creates long erotic foreplay, but it also requires preparation with plastic sheeting, especially if you choose to take the fun away from the bathroom.

Heighten The Senses

If this is your first experience into food play, cover your partner's hot spots with sweet treats before licking the area clean. Use angel delight during oral sex, which will also provide adequate calories. Some couples love to pie each other, while others enjoy the humiliation of being covered in food. Whatever food you choose to use, create a memorable session and burn off the additional calories through oral sex, foreplay, and hot sex. If you are a patient lover, lick the body clean before covering another part of your partner's anatomy. Food can easily turn a boring sixty-nine position into a wet and wild messy scene.

Phone Sex: The aim of this foreplay technique is to entice your partner into masturbation. It is easy to slip into role-play during a conversation over the phone. If it feels strange to describe dirty phrases to your partner to create his/her arousal, now is the time to experiment.

Although phone sex requires confidence, it has its benefits, one of which is to help you step into the role of a different person—your favorite actor/actress perhaps, or a confident dominatrix whose sole purpose is to turn on her client. If you feel a little nervous, write out a script beforehand and practice. This foreplay method could prove difficult for shy individuals who have not yet ventured out of his/her safe sexual environment. However, for other couples, phone sex will feel natural.

Phone sex has its spontaneous elements. It is easy to spring a surprising "dirty" phone call on your partner at any time of the day. If your partner phones you while you are driving, ignore the call. In the UK, if caught using a mobile phone, three points are added to the license, plus there is an additional fine.

During phone sex, lower your normal tone of voice to a sexier pitch, and imagine how your partner will react when you describe your fantasy in detail. Also think about how you are going to react to his/her words during phone sex. Will you strip off your clothes and masturbate, while listening to the deep fervent moans on the other end, or will you invoke the power of your sexual mind and describe a fantasy you would love to play out in reality.

Decide to step into a fantasy during phone sex and your sexual mind becomes alert and focused on arousal. Phone sex is wonderful as it opens the mind to its true potential. If you are wondering how to initiate sexy conversation, here are some examples:

- o "Can I tell you a secret? I am wearing no underwear under my skirt? Are you ready to turn me juicy?"
- o "I'm horny. Would you pounce on me if I were stood before you naked?"
- o "Strip off your clothes. I want to go down on you?"
- o "Baby, I want you to tie me up and dominate me right now."

Heighten The Senses

Imagine a sexual fantasy. Does your partner have a secret crush on a famous actor/actress? If so, it's time to step into that role and play the part. Does s/he have an accent or appear dominant in reality? Does your partner's fantasy figure create excitement in your genitals? Rid the mind of insecurities and imagine that you have become the character of your partner's dreams. Moan, masturbate, and excite your partner with saucy details of your solo masturbation session throughout phone sex.

Shower Sex: This method of foreplay allows you to get kinky and clean with your partner at the same time. For once, forget about your body hang ups by diminishing your ego—the part of your mind, which states you are fat, ugly, old, or embarrassed. Now, imagine a white light full of confidence, and step into it.

During shower sex, experiment with oral sex, or use the spray nozzle of the shower to stimulate your partner's genitals. Do you crave experimental sex or a sensation that feels extraordinarily different? Rim your partner's ass with your tongue to create variety. This is an especially powerful move when performed on a man.

A favorite move I like to request from a partner is for him to lather a sponge and wash my body and hair. It feels erotic to give a partner free reign over my hygiene. Cover your bodies in foam and share a deep French kiss.

Heighten The Senses

Have you had enough of performing oral sex and sharing hot passionate kisses in the shower? If so, try shower sex. This move requires trust, stamina, and relaxation in both the mind and body. It is difficult to use a condom in the shower therefore teamwork is necessary. Water turns the area slippery, which creates a struggle to remain still throughout sexual intercourse. Using a condom is also difficult, so ensure that your partner is free of sexually transmitted diseases (STDs). To have comfortable shower sex, you must be heavily lubricated to allow his penis to slip in and out. Build up a good rhythm with your partner. If you are not a fan of oral sex because of its scent and taste, there is no excuse when you take a shower together. Perform oral sex on your partner, while he holds the showerhead directly over your head. This is difficult. Water enters the nose, streams over your eyes, and makes it difficult to concentrate on the act. If it feels more comfortable giving oral sex without the added pressure of water stealing your focus, ask your partner to lie down in the bath or shower (if large enough). Alternatively, turn off the shower and conclude your rendezvous in the bedroom.

Cybersex: Similar to phone sex, except cybersex allows you to act out the fantasy online. Become the character of your partner's dreams. Many couples meet online, where a relationship then develops. Shy individuals may prefer online dating to socializing with friends, and many seek a kind, compassionate partner who brings out the best in his/her personality.

Many new mobile phone designs allow both Internet and email access, so now it is easier to log into your social networking account and begin a stimulating conversation with your partner. Cybersex can take place anywhere you have Internet access. It adds a fun element to any boring workday.

Cybersex allows you to become a sexually exciting woman. A shy female can turn into a dominatrix if she has the confidence to step into character. To further surprise a partner, take a naughty picture of your fingers wrapped around your breasts/penis, and send it to your partner.

If you are quite conservative, it may feel alien to unleash a sexual side. However, if you do, it gives your partner the opportunity to view you in a new light. Continue cybersex with your partner or potential love interest, and the next time you meet, your mind will remember every second of the exciting foreplay. To initiate cybersex, use these examples:

- o "What would you say if I told you I was naked and masturbating right now? Does that turn you on?"
- o "I can't wait to get my hands on you."
- o "Can I cover you in oil, and run my nipples around your lips?"
- o "My lips are fully fixed around your dick. Tell me how hard you are right now."

Heighten The Senses

Cybersex is an exciting form of foreplay, which can be performed anywhere you have Internet access. However, for some couples, it could grow boring. An interesting but spontaneous scene would be to set up a cybersex date. During my last online relationship, I enjoyed turning on my partner while he was at work. If you find it difficult to display a spontaneous side, set your preferred date. Do you choose a rainstorm, posh hotel, or two strangers who meet in odd circumstances? Set the scene, and imagine how you would react in that fantasy. Would you act differently from your usual personality? If you are normally shy or reserved in the bedroom, will a dot of cybersex unleash a newfound spontaneous side? Play out your ideal fantasy to drive your partner crazy.

Ice: This wonderful tool creates a one of a kind sensation on the skin. Ice arouses every nerve ending in the body. Tease an ice cube down your partner's neck, breasts, and around each nipple. Dribble the ice cube beyond your partner's hips, and watch for a reaction. Add the warm breath of a kiss over the tingly areas to drive her crazy.

Heighten The Senses

Blindfold your partner, and lie him/her face down on the bed, sofa, or massage table. Tease an ice cube down the spine, circle it around the lower back, and rub it over the backs of the knees, calves, and thighs. If you want to keep your partner up all night pining for your touch, use ice to your advantage. When the ice melts, use your warm tongue to add a varied sensation to your partner's spine and surrounding areas. Turn him/her into a writhing horny devil. Ice always creates a memorable session.

Massage: This move feels great when performed over a naked, semi-naked, or fully clothed body. Add essential oils to carrier oil and mix well before rubbing it into your partner's body to relax or stimulate his/her nervous system. Edible massage oils are ideal if you fancy stimulating the body with your tongue, rather than the hands.

Perform a full body massage on your partner, and rub in the essence vigorously. The silky feeling upon the skin is sexy for both the provider and lucky receiver. Massage incorporates the important element of touch, and creates desire in your partner. Full body massages can take over an hour. Before the start of the massage, scan your partner's body for tense muscles. Stress is often felt in the shoulders and lower back.

Heighten The Senses

Gently brush the fingertips or a feather over your partner's skin. The slight sensation sets alight every nerve ending in the body. Massage expertise is not necessary, as fingertip stroking will create incredible delight in your partner's mind, causing your pleasure. The one on the receiving end of this relaxing foreplay will grow horny. Let the waves of pleasure envelop your mind and body, and sex will slip to the forefront of your mind. Add oil to the body with firm strokes, and continue with the massage to build strong excitement in your partner. Climb on top of your partner, and slide over his/her oily body, while running your nails into his/her scalp to build pleasurable ambiance.

Text Sex: Similar to phone and cybersex, but text sex allows you to host the fantasy using your mobile phone through dirty phrases to arouse your partner. Text sex is a spontaneous foreplay move. Entice your partner with filthy words at any time of the day, and your true sexual power will shine through. Surprise your partner at work or while he's out with his friends to turn his thoughts onto you.

Avoid sending an explicit text if you know your partner is driving. Using a mobile phone at the wheel is dangerous and could cause serious accidents, injury, and death to yourself and others. If you have no idea of what to write, here are some samples:

- "I'm desperate to get my hands on you right now."
- "Bet you can't guess what was going through my kinky mind during my boring afternoon meeting?"
- "You, me, and a bottle of baby oil tonight."
- "Thinking about you starring in my fantasy is driving me nuts for you."
- "Don't forget the whipped cream tonight, sexy. Your dick is getting covered."
- "Bet you'd love to put your mouth where my hand is right now."

Heighten The Senses

Write a dirty text and send it to your partner when you know that s/he is busy at work. Text sex is a fun tool, which distracts your partner's concentration away from the unhealthy stress of deadlines. This is positive. Visualize a horny image or masturbation fantasy. Set your partner's mind racing with explicit words. Avoid sending an explicit text if you know your partner is driving. Choose text sex as the perfect way to turn on your partner's sexual mind. If your partner is out with his friends, entice him with horny messages. Soon enough, your partner's mind will be on red alert waiting for another randy message from you.

Bathing: If you have a large tub, sex in the bath is worthwhile—although it could turn a little wet and messy. Add three drops each of essential oil of sandalwood, vanilla, and lavender to the bathtub. These oils soothe the nervous system and perfume the air.

If you have the space for romantic elements, light a couple of scented candles or incense, and dim the lights to turn the scene sexual. Be careful not to slip in the bath, especially with the added essential oils.

Lie on top of your partner in between his/her legs. If the bath is large enough, sit opposite your partner. In addition, when the body is relaxed and content, the sexual mind resurfaces.

Heighten The Senses

Heighten the visual and auditory senses with dirty words whispered beside his/her ear. Alternatively, stimulate your partner's scalp with your nails. Open your mind to your present surroundings—the sound of flickering candles (if used), your partner's breaths, or the gentle waves of the water. Wash your partner's hair slowly and massage the scalp. When two naked bodies rub together, the mind is forced to reminisce about the early days of romance. Sex in the bath must be gentle and synchronized to prevent the water from sloshing everywhere.

The Moaning Kiss: The lips are one of the most sensual erogenous zones in the body. A multitude of pleasures are felt during a moaning kiss. During an orgasm, signal your excitement by moaning in your partner's mouth. S/he may feel a slight tingle running down the spine, or goose bumps all over the skin. The moaning kiss is perfect to incorporate into many of the preceding foreplay methods, i.e. shower sex and domination etc.

Heighten The Senses

Blindfold your partner, tie up the hands, and rub your genitals across your partner's chest. Move to his/her mouth to plant a passionate moaning kiss that does a little more than set fireworks to the genitals. Masturbate your partner until s/he gives you a reciprocal moaning kiss.

Water Sports: Not every couple enjoys the pleasure of water sports, also known as golden showers—urinating on a partner. The scent of urine is stronger in some individuals and is dependent on the food/drinks consumed. Some foods like fish and asparagus can affect the scent of urine, so these are best avoided if you plan to dabble in water sports.

Experimenting with water sports is both adventurous and kinky. Contrary to what society states, urine is over ninety percent sterile, plus it is a wonderful anti-aging moisturizer for the skin.[46] It heals the body internally through the re-absorption of vitamins, minerals, and essential nutrients. Urea—an extract of urine—is often added to many expensive anti-aging products.[47]

Heighten The Senses

Urinate on your partner while taking a shower together. Even if you cover only the back or the legs, experiment with water sports. If you feel adventurous, sit on your partner's face, cover it in urine, then share a passionate kiss. Lay a plastic sheet on the bed and experiment away from the shower. Unbelievably, the essential nutrients found in urine are re-absorbed into the skin. Urine does not scent the skin, but it does contain natural pheromones. It is healing and a natural by product of the body. It is a wonderful softening skin tonic, but water sports will not suit everyone.

Warning: Be prepared for a messy scene if you choose to experiment away from the shower.

GET IN SEXY SHAPE

SEXUAL WORKOUTS

Regular sex is a fantastic way to tone the body, boost the immune system, and relieve stress through the emission of endorphins. Girl-on-top and reverse cowgirl positions are two of the best buttock workouts for women. Other positions detailed in this chapter are a little more tougher than average because they require stamina and upper body strength.

Exercise of any kind, including sex, kissing, oral sex, and foreplay, all work to increase your levels of endurance. Here is a quick summary of my ten favorite sexual positions and four variations of each, except for missionary, which contains seven variations.

1. **Missionary**: This is the most basic of lovemaking positions for couples. It is easy to kiss during missionary, and many women prefer it to the more difficult experimental positions e.g. opposite ends or standing sex. Although missionary sex does not offer a dynamic thigh and buttock workout, there are seven variations included in this chapter to stimulate your inventive side.

2. **Doggy Style**: If you enjoy deep penetrative sex, this position satisfies the female g-spot. The buttocks play a starring role, seducing your partner, and most men enjoy a pair of peachy buttocks to grab onto. Incorporate gentle spanking into role-play, if you both love kinky sex. This position is also ideal for men who are a little smaller than average in the trouser department. With the buttocks spread, the skin looks and feels tighter, so there is no need to worry about visible fat or cellulite.

3. **Girl-On-Top**: The ideal position for confident women to show off their figures, display sexual prowess, and take control of a partner. Girl-on-top tones the inner thigh and buttock muscles, especially when performed consistently. Show off a confident side by seducing your partner, and give him a memory or two to reminisce over. When the thighs fatigue—which they will after a short period—thrust slowly to build up your

energy reserves. This position requires self-confidence, stamina, and a love for experimental sex.

4. **Reverse Cowgirl**: If you have self-confidence, stamina, and enthusiasm, you will love reverse cowgirl. This position tones the buttocks, and also gives your partner a great view. Masturbate easily during performance of this position, and control the depth of penetration. If your sole aim is to give your partner a memorable sex session by pushing him to the brink of orgasm, reverse cowgirl will work wonders!

5. **Spoons**: This position is ideal for morning sex when you are both half asleep, but feeling horny. It gives you the chance to cuddle your partner and make love. Ask your partner to gently bite the nape of your neck and/or suck on your sensitive earlobes to send wonderful sensations to the genitals.

6. **Seated Sex**: This position works effectively to tone and shape the muscles of the thighs and buttocks. It also offers deep penetration as well as providing easy access to stimulate the clitoris with fingers or toys. Arouse your partner's testicles and g-spot with a massage from your thumb and forefinger. Encourage your partner to lick up and down your spine, lean back, and transfer his hands onto your breasts.

7. **Press-Up Sex**: If you love raunchy positions that require strength, stamina, and deep penetration, you have to try press-up sex. Show off your figure, work the arms, and test your mental strength. Rest your ankles on the bed, and ask your partner to climb on top and penetrate you. If you have a good level of fitness, press-up sex will still be challenging, but at least you'll be able to experiment for a couple of minutes or longer, if super fit. Press-up sex gets the heart pumping, creates intimacy, and provides a wonderful resistance type workout to tone the female body.

8. **Upside Down Sex**: I am not relating to the wheelbarrow or handstand, as even I struggle with those two positions. Upside down sex requires your partner to hold you firmly, while your upper body hangs off the bed. Men require strong upper body strength, and women require substantial abdominal strength to remain in position without discomfort. The rush of blood to the head heightens every nerve ending in the body.

9. **Standing Sex**: A great position, which is perfect to trial as a quickie. Unless you have athletic strength, it is impossible to conduct usual foreplay or have sex for hours. However, if you cut out the foreplay or

experiment with foreplay beforehand, standing sex feels raunchy. Men require a good level of upper body strength and stamina to hold a partner in position and make love satisfactory.

10. **Opposite Ends**: Lie on top of your partner, but remain at opposite ends. This position requires flexibility in the thighs, a good rhythm, and excellent effort from the thigh and buttocks. Give your partner a show he will never forget by masturbating. Alternatively, allow him to use a vibrator on your hot spot to bring you to a fulfilling orgasm. Although this position may not look easy, practice makes perfect. If you experiment regularly, your thighs will gain in strength, but you should expect muscular aches afterward.

Missionary Sex: Position 1

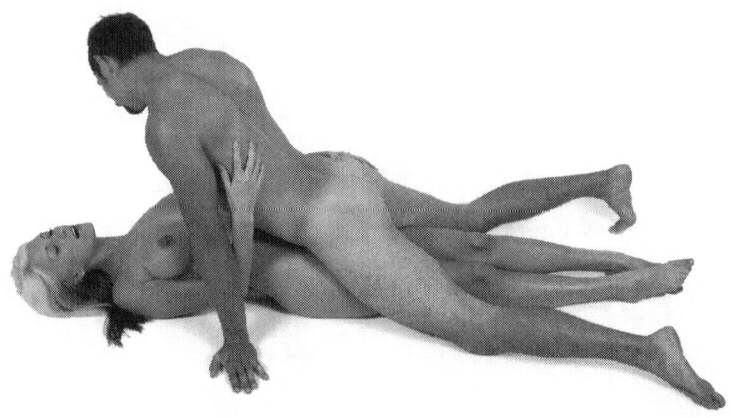

Positives:

- This is the most basic of missionary positions enjoyed by a huge variety of men/women.
- It creates a sensual lovemaking scene.
- A couple can experiment with long erotic kisses, while the bodies bump and grind to delicious orgasms.
- It is easy for a woman to return thrust, which tones the buttock and thigh muscles.
- Grip your partner's buttocks and moan beside his ear to stimulate his nerve endings.
- If you have long nails or extensions, run your nails down his back to heighten his arousal.

Negatives:

- It could feel quite limiting for a woman.
- This position fails to stimulate the clitoris, unless you indulge in foreplay before sexual penetration.
- This position can grow boring, especially if it is repeatedly entertained.
- Unfit women may find it difficult to return thrust. Therefore, it may not offer much of a workout to the thigh and buttock areas.

Missionary Sex: Position 2

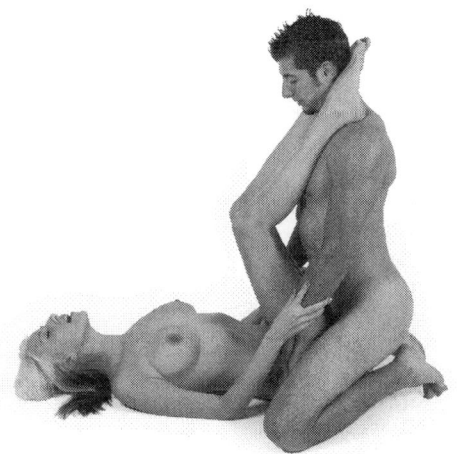

Positives:

- This missionary position stimulates the g-spot easily.
- Confidently display your breasts, and allow your partner to view your face reacting to his horny thrusts.
- Talk filthy, moan, and reach up to run your fingers through his chest hair.
- Indulge in passionate kisses if your legs are flexible enough to bend rearward.

Negatives:

- Unless you are already flexible, this position creates difficulty for couples to kiss.
- Women with body hang-ups may struggle to display their figures confidently.
- This enhanced missionary position provides deeper penetration than basic legs down missionary sex. Therefore, it is not ideal if you hate g-spot stimulation.

Missionary Sex: Position 3

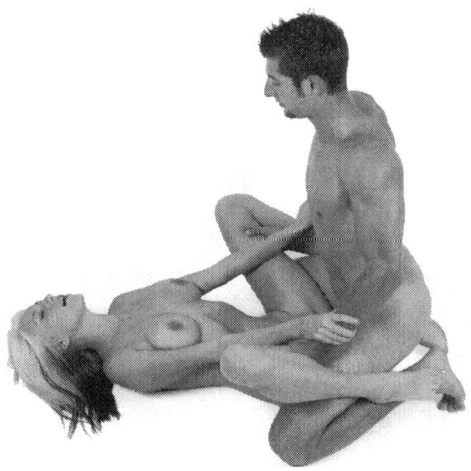

Positives:

- Make intense eye contact with your partner during deep penetration.
- This position will force ardent moans to roll off your tongue.
- Before sex, allow your partner to stimulate your clitoris with his penis, fingers, or a sex toy.
- This position instantly flattens the abdominals.
- Stroke his legs with your fingers and/or nails, or massage his balls if you are able to reach.
- Create intimacy by pulling your partner onto you and wrapping your leg around his hips.

Negatives:

- Erotic kisses could divert his attention away from clitoral stimulation.
- Confidence is required. Not every woman likes to display the "orgasm" face via expressions and moans.
- Requires flexibility in the upper body and legs to kiss comfortably.
- This position may not appeal to women who hate deep penetration.

Missionary Sex Position 4

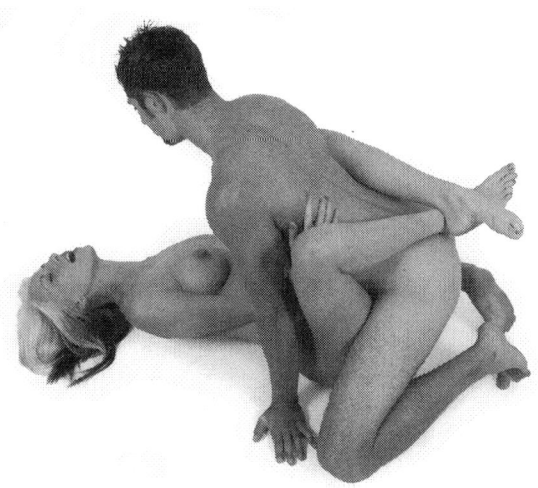

Positives:

- Satisfies the female g-spot.
- Wrap your legs around your partner and squeeze the thighs to tone the inner thigh area.
- Display enthusiasm with moans, explicit words, and flirty facial gestures.
- Allow his penis to slip out occasionally to stroke your clitoris.
- It's easy to passionately embrace in this position.

Negatives:

- The thighs will fatigue if you continuously return thrust.
- Displaying the upper half of your figure requires confidence.
- Requires flexibility in the inner thigh to remain in position, return thrust, and prevent muscle fatigue.
- Close the eyes if the thought of your partner viewing your "orgasm" face turns you anxious.

Missionary Sex: Position 5

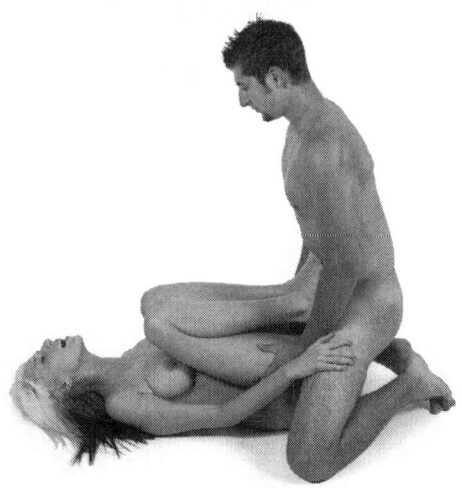

Positives:

- This position provides deep penetration through g-spot stimulation.
- Display your facial pleasure and beautiful breasts during intercourse.
- If you can reach, give his ass a good squeeze during penetration.
- The legs cover the abdominals. In addition, pulling in the legs tightens the buttocks.
- Run your fingertips or nails over his chest or thigh area to stimulate his nerve endings.
- Your ass will get a thorough workout if you return thrust.

Negatives:

- A degree of fitness is required to continuously meet his thrust.
- With additional effort, your thighs could start to ache or turn numb.
- The wider gap between you could create difficulty in kissing.
- This position does not provide enough direct stimulation to the clitoris.

Missionary Sex: Position 6

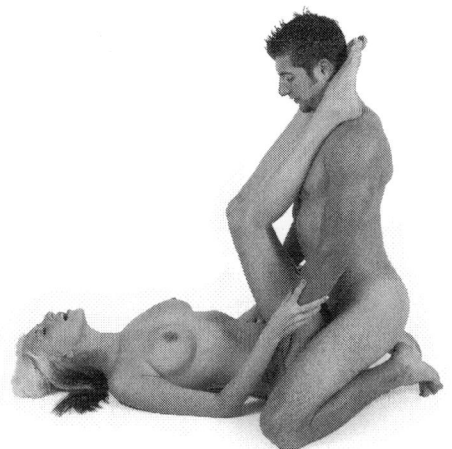

Positives:

- Give the buttocks a thorough workout by matching each of your partner's thrusts.
- Satisfies the female g-spot, which can cause some women to multi-orgasm.
- Titillate your partner through deep moans and explicit conversation.
- The legs partially cover the abdominals; perfect if you are shy about displaying the upper half of your figure.
- Although it does not provide direct clitoral stimulation, your fingers are free to masturbate. Alternatively, reach down and tickle his testicles.

Negatives:

- Not the ideal position for women who dislike deep g-spot stimulation.
- A general level of fitness is required to return thrust.
- This position provides intense sex without the erotic element of deep passionate kisses.

Missionary Sex: Position 7

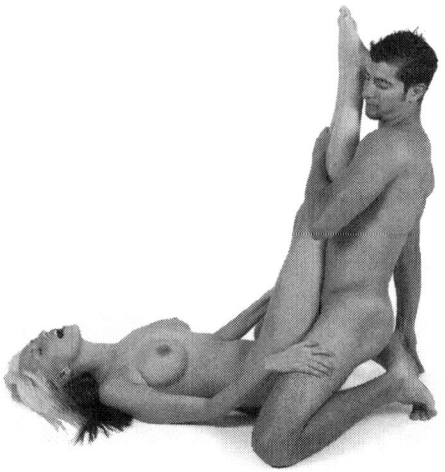

Positives:

- You have the opportunity to thrust as hard as you like, while he grips your legs.
- Vary the pressure; penetrate slow or faster dependent on the current mood of you and that of your partner.
- Your breasts, elegant neck, and "orgasm" face is on show. Use them to your advantage.
- Give him the perfect view of your bouncing breasts, while he holds and strokes your legs. To create his further excitement, push your breasts together and titillate the nipples.

Negatives

- This position makes it impossible to kiss passionately.
- This missionary position requires bodily confidence to display your upper body and "orgasm" face.
- If you dislike deep vaginal penetration, avoid this position and stick to basic missionary.

Doggy Style: Position 1

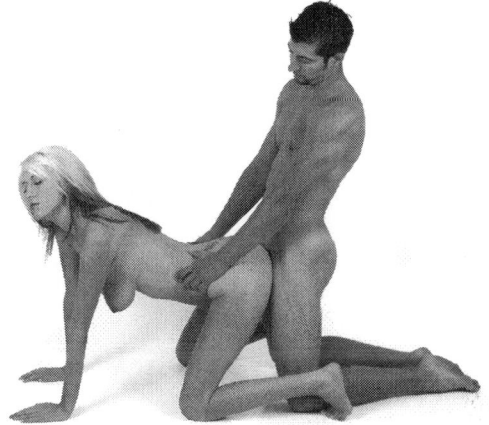

Positives:

- This bent over position "tightens" the buttocks.
- Continuously return thrust to work the buttock muscles.
- This position encourages a healthy toxin-cleansing sweat.
- Displays the perfect outline of your curves.
- This position provides deep g-spot stimulation.
- Allow your partner to spank or massage your buttocks during sex.
- You have free reign to stroke your clitoris.
- Fondle his testicles with your fingers or a sex toy.

Negatives:

- Does not have the romantic elements of missionary.
- This position makes it difficult to comfortably kiss.
- Offers deep g-spot stimulation. If your partner's penis is large it could create discomfort.
- Doggy style sex is deemed as mischievous sex rather than sensual lovemaking.

Doggy Style: Position 2

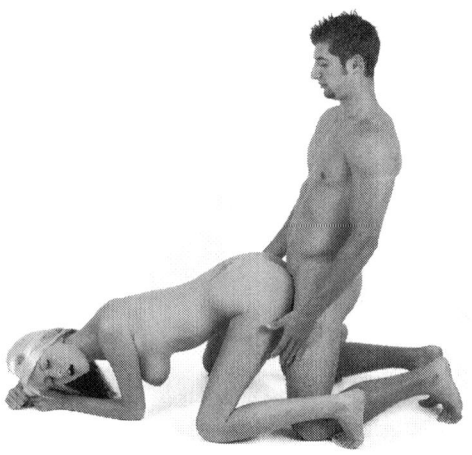

Positives:

- Satisfies the female g-spot.
- The buttocks appear toned, and the curves of the female figure provide visual satisfaction for your partner.
- You can tone the buttocks with return thrusts.
- Stroke the clitoris together, or request that he massages your buttocks while you masturbate.

Negatives:

- This position does not create the simplicity to embrace.
- Deep g-spot stimulation could feel uncomfortable for many women.
- Bodily confidence is required.
- It may not appeal to couples who enjoy intimacy and kissing.

Doggy Style: Position 3

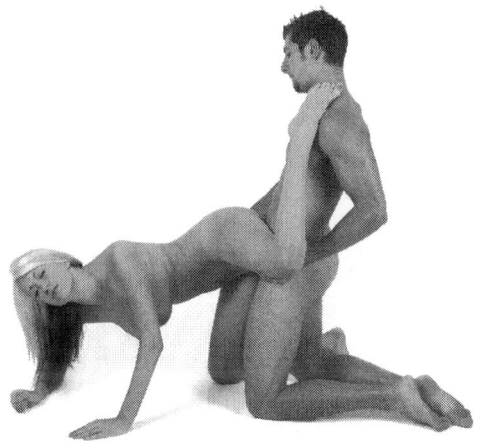

Positives:

- This position tones the muscles of the arms when practiced regularly
- Balance is essential in order to remain upright.
- Could create multi-orgasmic pleasure in women.
- Determined effort will ensure that the thigh and buttock muscles get a thorough workout.

Negatives:

- This position requires balance and focus, therefore it may be difficult to maintain for long periods.
- No opportunity to masturbate.
- Requires strength in the upper body.
- The difficult positioning could cause the penis to slide out several times.
- This position provides no opportunity to embrace.
- Will tire the thigh and buttock muscles after a relatively short period.

Doggy Style: Position 4

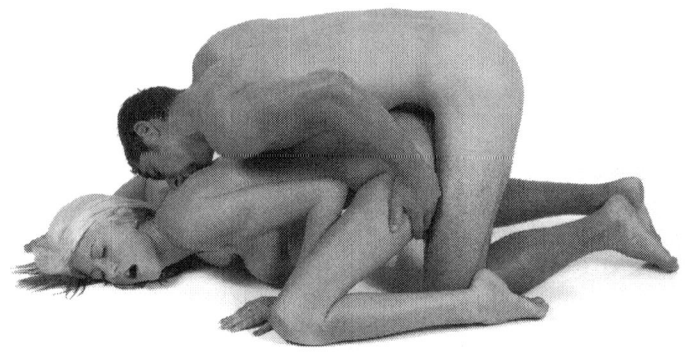

Positives:

- Your partner can stimulate the nape of your neck, squeeze your buttocks, and lick up and down your spine.
- Although difficult, it may be possible to kiss in this position.
- Provides a deep level of intimacy.
- He can easy access to your clitoris.
- Tickle his testicles with your fingers or a sex toy.

Negatives:

- If you prefer an easy position in which to embrace, this position may not be for you.
- If your partner has a large member, it will stimulate the g-spot and create discomfort in many women.
- It may be difficult to focus on a clitoral orgasm.

Girl-on-Top: Position 1

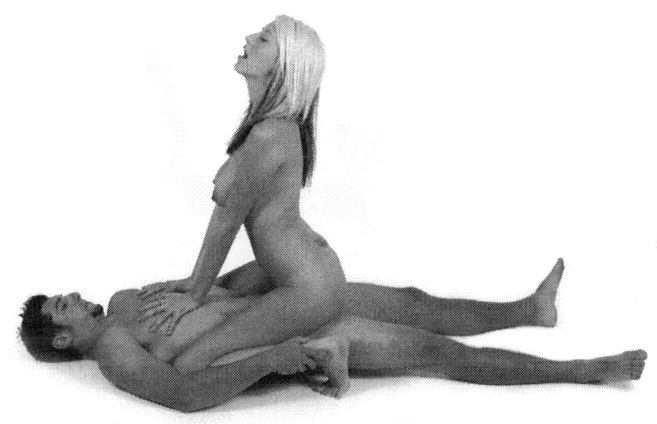

Positives:

- The ideal position for confident women to show off their stamina and bedroom skills.
- Sex on top uses the muscles of the thighs and buttocks—giving them a thorough workout.
- Tie up his hands and dominate him. Alternatively, rub your hands or nails up and down his chest to heighten his senses.
- You can make love slowly, while kissing passionately.
- Masturbate to excite him visually.
- It is easy to control the depth of pressure during lovemaking, especially when the thighs feel fatigued.
- Massage your breasts and nipples, or dangle them over his mouth while his hands are tied.

Negatives:

- It requires a good level of fitness in the buttocks and thigh muscles.
- If you continue with this position for over half an hour, the thighs and buttocks will ache afterward.
- Not an ideal position for shy women who feel body conscious.

Girl-on-Top: Position 2

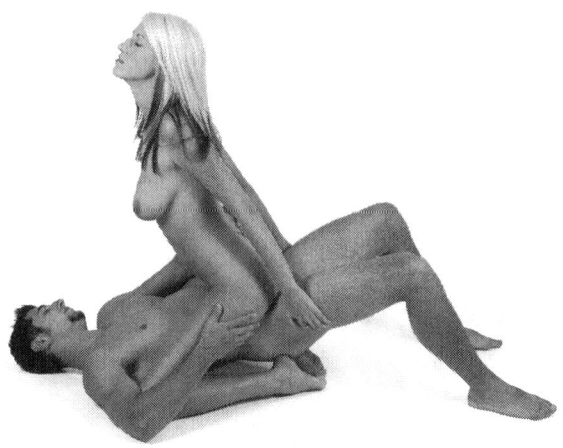

Positives:

- Lean forward slightly to display your beautiful bouncing breasts.
- If he raises his knees, it creates further comfort for you to thrust.
- He can stimulate your breasts, admire your pleasure, and stroke your thighs, breasts and nipples during lovemaking.
- Tickle his testicles to heighten his pleasure.
- The clitoris is within easy reach. Let your partner stroke you to ecstasy, or give him a memorable view of you masturbating.
- Practice slow and fast thrusts to carry your partner to the brink of ecstasy.
- Rest your legs underneath his buttocks in the lotus position to achieve good balance. When practiced regularly, this position tones the thighs.

Negatives:

- It may be difficult to focus on your orgasm during masturbation.
- This position requires stamina, enthusiasm, and bodily confidence.
- In the lotus position, thigh strength and flexibility is required to thrust. Therefore, it may cause an ache a day or two afterward.

Girl-on-Top: Position 3

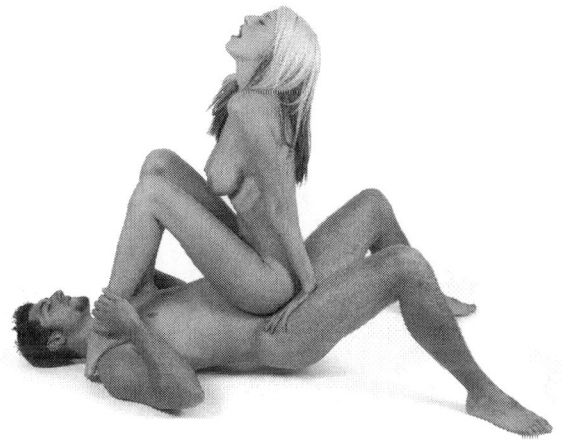

Positives:

- Provides a great view of his penis slipping in and out during lovemaking.
- While you put in the effort to thrust, he has easy access to your clitoris.
- It is easy to control the depth of pressure throughout sex.
- If you have strong upper body strength, try to balance on one hand. Use the other free hand to massage his testicles and perineum. Alternatively, titillate his mind into mutual masturbation.

Negatives:

- Balancing on your partner's thighs could create his discomfort.
- Arm, thigh, and buttock strength is required to make love comfortably.
- This position requires bodily confidence.
- Requires flexibility to lean forward and embrace.

Girl-on-Top: Position 4

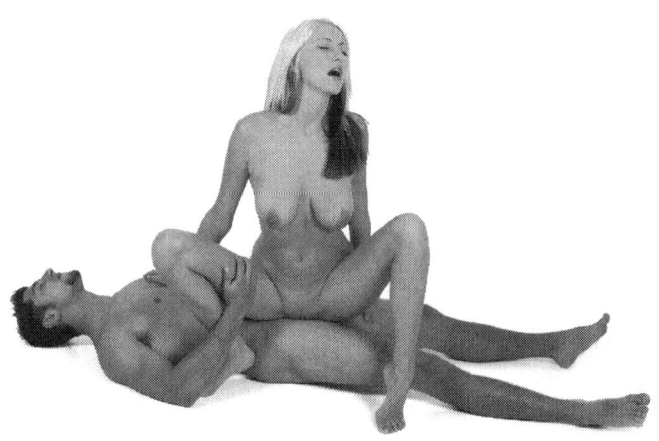

Positives:

- With exerted effort, this position gives the buttock and thigh areas a superb workout.
- Pull in the stomach to appear slimmer. This position is exciting for your partner, as he has the visual delight of your buttocks slapping up and down on his penis.
- He has easy access to fondle your clitoris and breasts.

Negatives:

- This position requires thigh and arm strength.
- It is difficult to embrace in this raunchy position.
- Leaning on his thighs during lovemaking could create his discomfort.
- If you put in consistent effort, there will be muscular aches afterward.
- Women require a general level of stamina.

Reverse Cowgirl: Position 1

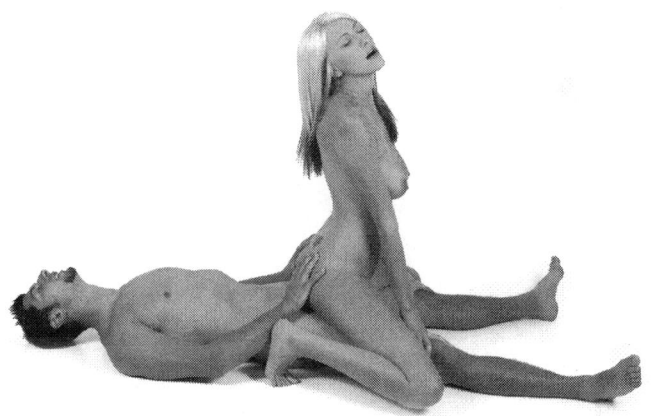

Positives:

- This position offers deep g-spot penetration to create multi-orgasms.
- Stroke his legs, and lean forward to give him a great view of him slipping in and out, while you stroke his legs and massage his feet.
- Tickle his testicles with your fingers or a vibrating sex toy to give him a unique sensation.
- Control the thrusts with ease when the legs fatigue.
- You have easy access to stroke your clitoris.
- In this position, the buttocks look tighter.
- The ideal position to arouse male buttock enthusiasts.

Negatives:

- It may be difficult for shy or non-experimental women to maintain.
- Requires stamina in the buttocks and thighs to maintain this position for longer periods.
- A larger than average penis could create discomfort for some women.
- It may be difficult to kiss.

Reverse Cowgirl: Position 2

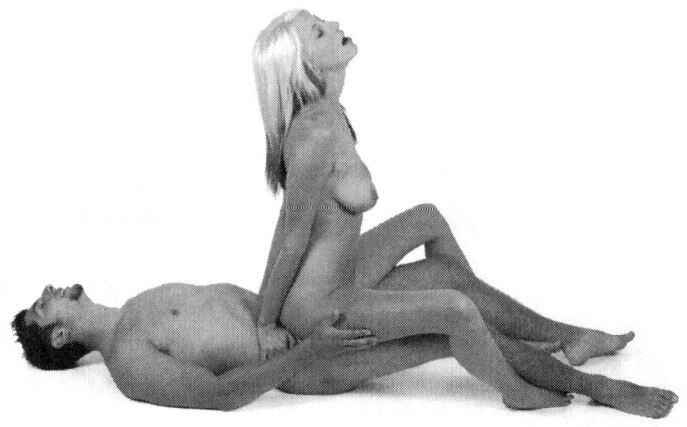

Positives:

- Tones the buttocks and thigh areas.
- Give your partner a great view of your ass thrashing him relentlessly.
- Offers deep vaginal penetration—perfect to cause multi-orgasms.
- Allow your partner to squeeze your buttocks with every thrust and even stroke your clitoris with a little effort.
- Builds up a deep detoxifying sweat.
- Provides the opportunity to slow the thrusts when the muscles in the thighs start to burn.
- He can run his nails up and down your spine to tease your nerve endings.
- Displays the gorgeous curves of your body.

Negatives:

- Your partner will be unable to view you masturbating.
- Unless he has very long arms, it may be difficult for him to reach around to stimulate your clitoris.
- He is unable to view your facial pleasures.
- A general level of fitness is necessary.

Reverse Cowgirl: Position 3

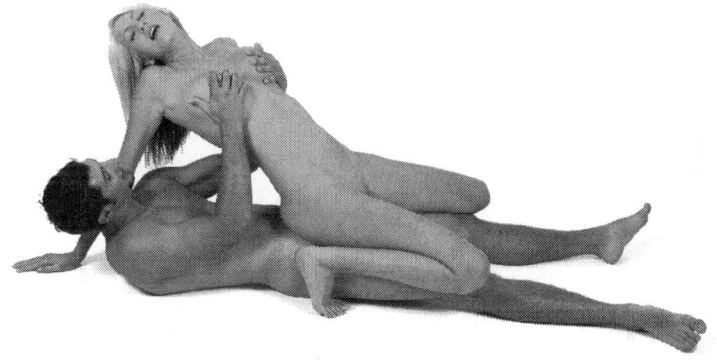

Positives:

- Give him a wonderful view of your curves while making tender love.
- Stimulate your clitoris alone, or mutually masturbate with your partner.
- He can fondle your breasts, while you work your thighs and buttocks. Allow him to squeeze the flesh of your buttocks, or request that he excites your spine.
- If performed regularly, the thigh and buttock muscles will start to tone.

Negatives:

- This position could make it tiresome for women with no general level of fitness.
- Difficult to kiss.
- Upper body strength is required to remain comfortable.
- Will cause an ache in both the thighs and buttocks muscles.
- If you lean on your partner for balance, it could create his discomfort.
- Requires substantial thigh strength to thrust in this position.

Reverse Cowgirl: Position 4

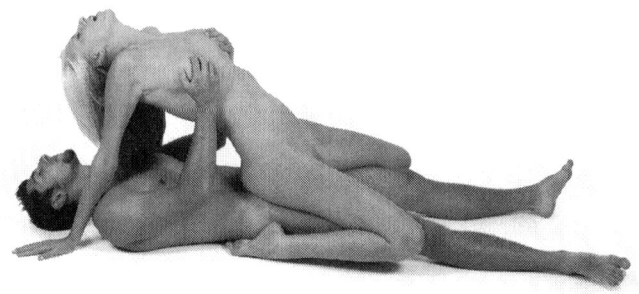

Positives:

- Lean back fully on your partner, and allow him easy access to fondle your breasts. If he can reach round he could also stimulate your clitoris.
- Provides the opportunity to mutually stroke your clitoris.
- This position gives you the chance to show off your incredible stamina and lovemaking skills.
- Provides a synchronistic workout for the thighs, buttocks, and arms.
- Allows the opportunity to kiss.

Negatives:

- Quite a difficult position in which to continuously thrust. Work on building leg strength and stamina in the gym with weight training, or try performing lunges and squats at home.
- The thigh and buttocks may fatigue easily, and the continuous method may cause an ache a day or two afterward.
- It may be difficult to balance on one hand, continually make love to your partner, and stroke the clitoris at the same time.
- The kiss may not feel as passionate as it would feel face to face.

Spoons: Position 1

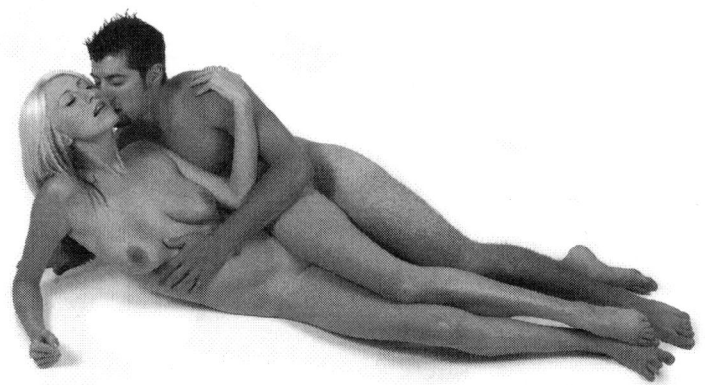

Positives:

- Provides easy access for your partner to stroke your breasts.
- This position allows you to mutually masturbate together.
- Wake up your partner by licking up and down her spine.
- Experiment with long passionate kisses.
- It requires hardly any stamina and is the "lazy" lovemaking position for those who love it.

Negatives:

- Does not offer much of a full body workout.
- This effortless position will not burn many calories.
- If you do not return thrust, the thighs and buttocks will not achieve a thorough workout.
- Not the perfect position to wake up to if you dislike morning sex.

Spoons: Position 2

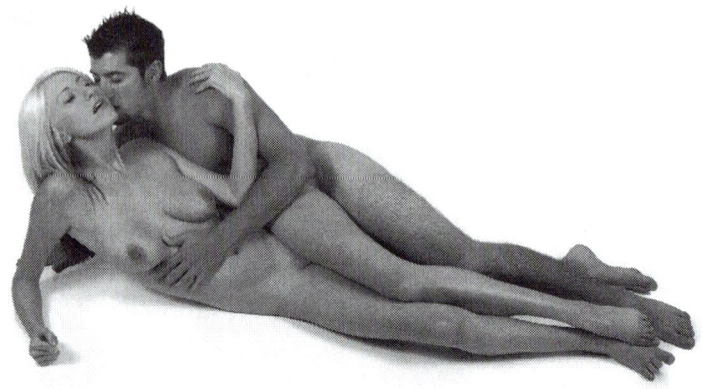

Positives:

- This position allows you both to get kinky while lay on a sofa or bed together.
- He can plant butterfly kisses on your elegant neck, or nibble your ears to stimulate your arousal.
- Provides various ways in how to reach orgasm.
- A comfortable yet intimate position that creates gratification.
- An intimate position where you can embrace and excite other areas of the body.

Negatives:

- It may not offer a thorough cardiovascular workout, which detoxifies the skin.
- This position may not burn many calories, nor does it offer a full body workout.

Spoons: Position 3

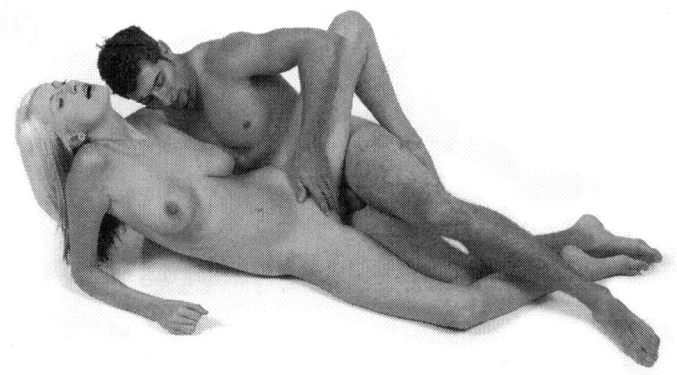

Positives:

- Share a passionate kiss, while he strokes you to orgasm.
- Allow him to watch you masturbate, while he grows visually excited.
- Massage your partner's testicles during penetration.
- Mutually masturbate together, or use a sex toy to reach climax.
- Give him easy access to lick and kiss the nape of your neck, behind your ears, and along your spine.

Negatives:

- If you prefer energetic thrusts during penetration, this "lazy" position does not provide much of a thorough workout.
- The thigh and buttock "problem" areas in women do not get a satisfying workout.
- Confidence is required, especially if you dislike telling or showing your partner how you like to be touched.

Spoons: Position 4

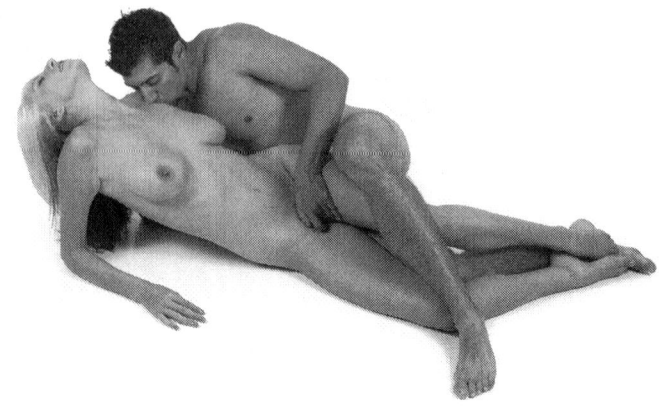

Positives:

- He can massage your breasts, kiss your nipples, and stroke your clitoris.
- This position is easy lovemaking and requires very little stamina.
- If you love slow lovemaking, this position will meet your needs.
- He can brush his lips over your skin to heighten your senses.
- The perfect position in which to dominate your partner.
- Share long erotic kisses.
- Allows for shallow or deeper penetration, dependent upon your sexual mood.

Negatives:

- It does not provide a thorough workout to the buttock and thighs.
- Lazy lovemaking.
- It may provide difficulty in teasing his genitals.

Seated Sex: Position 1

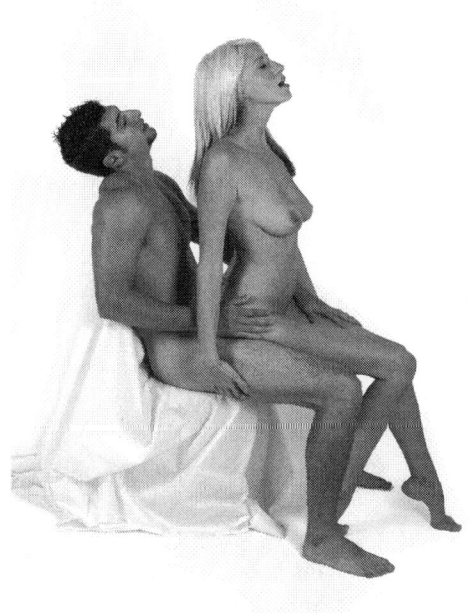

Positives:

- With substantial effort, this position tones the thigh and buttock areas.
- Control the depth of penetration easily when the thighs fatigue.
- Stimulate his testicles with your fingers, or use a sex toy.
- Rub your clitoris, or watch him stroke you to ecstasy.
- It tones the body and builds great stamina, especially when performed regularly.
- He has easy access to stimulate your spine, nape of the neck, and other hot erogenous zones with his fingers, lips, and tongue.

Negatives:

- Considered to be raunchier than the usual romantic lovemaking positions.
- It may be difficult to kiss during lovemaking.
- Requires a general level of fitness to continuously thrust. .
- The thigh and buttock muscles will fatigue easily.

Seated Sex: Position 2

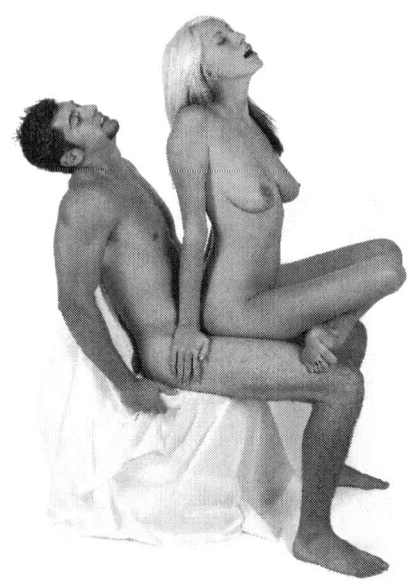

Positives:

- When performed regularly, this position tones the muscles of the arms, thighs, and buttocks.
- Could turn some women multi-orgasmic through deep penetration to the g-spot.
- He can fondle your breasts, spine, and neck during lovemaking.
- Offers a full body workout.

Negatives:

- Upper body strength and stamina is necessary in order to thrust continuously.
- Leaning on your partner for balance may create his discomfort.
- Expect muscular aches and discomfort one or two days afterward.

Seated Sex: Position 3

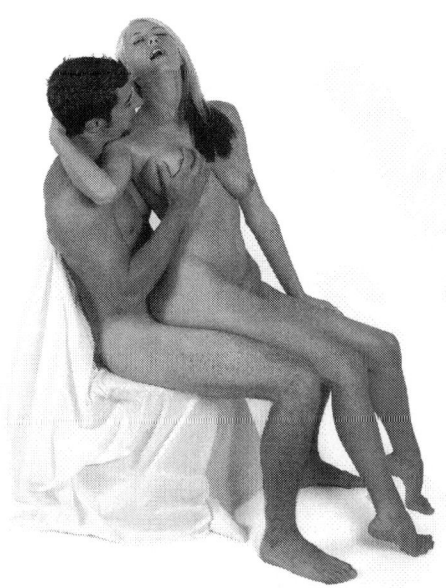

Positives:

- Provides him with easy access to your breasts and clitoris.
- You can masturbate alone or together, or give him full access to your clitoris, while you fully focus on your technique.
- This position builds stamina and causes thigh burn encouraging the metabolism to rise and burn off excess fat.
- G-spot stimulation can create a multi-orgasmic phase.

Negatives:

- If you dislike deep penetrative sex, this position could create discomfort.
- This position requires stamina and sufficient thigh and buttock strength.
- The thighs may fatigue after only a few minutes of lovemaking.
- It may be difficult to embrace throughout lovemaking.

Seated Sex: Position 4

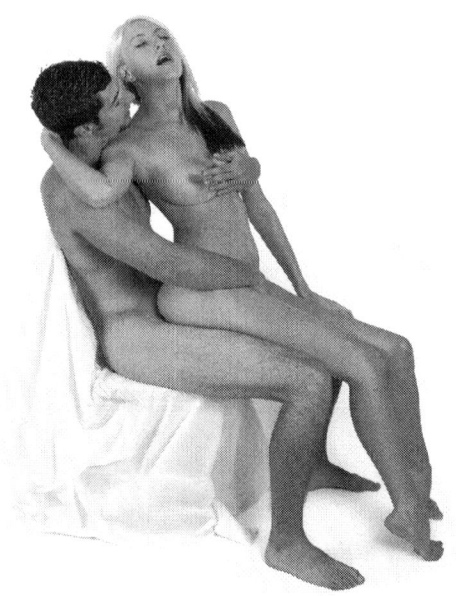

Positives:

- He has easy access to all your hot erogenous zones—clitoris, nape of the neck, and breasts.
- All the senses heighten with skin-on-skin contact, while he stimulates your erogenous zones.
- It is easy to control the depth of penetration.
- Reach simultaneous clitoral and g-spot orgasm during lovemaking.
- With effort, the thigh and buttock areas will appear more toned.

Negatives:

- Requires a good level of stamina.
- Focusing on your climax during lovemaking could be distracting.
- Could be tiresome to the thighs and cause an ache days afterward.

Press-Up Sex: Position 1

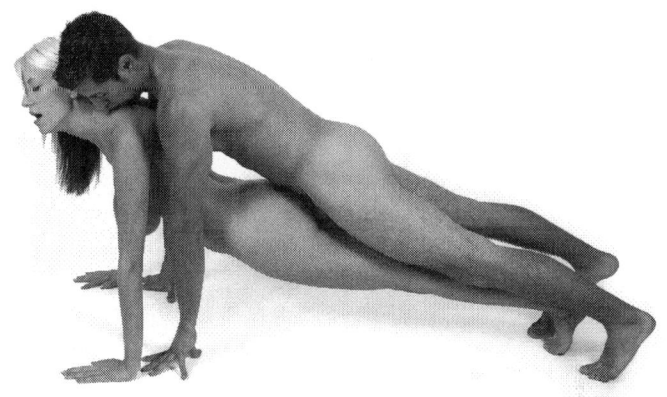

Positives:

- This position is ideal for experimental couples with excellent upper body strength.
- Provides a full body workout.
- Moan in her ear to create tingles down her spine.
- A great calorie-burning workout.
- He can kiss and nibble the nape of your neck during sex.
- Pulling in the abdominals strengthens this area, while you will tone the arms the longer you remain in position.
- Offers deep penetration similar to doggy style.

Negatives:

- This position requires upper body strength and a high degree of stamina.
- It will tire the body and arms after only a few minutes.
- If your partner is heavier than you, it could be difficult to maintain his bodyweight and make love comfortably.
- Does not allow for easy smooching.
- No room for clitoral stimulation or sensuous foreplay.

Press-Up Sex: Position 2

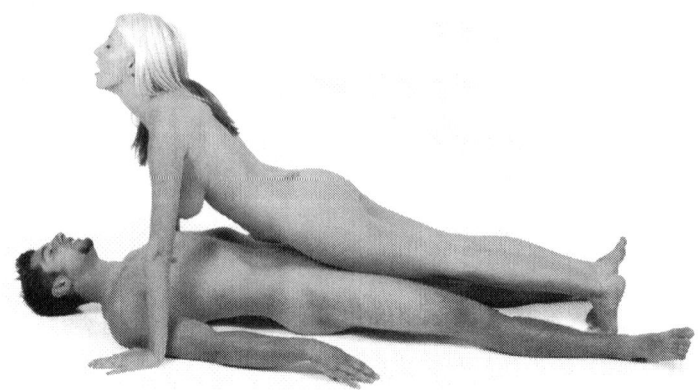

Positives:

- Display your bouncing breasts, while he encourages deep thrusts.
- This position tones the upper half of the body—a difficult to tone area in women.
- Offers the body a thorough workout, if you can maintain the position.
- If you love a sexually challenging workout, this is the perfect position for you.
- Requires enthusiasm and a positive mindset, especially when fatigue hits the arms.
- Builds a deep detoxifying sweat and burns calories.

Negatives:

- This position makes it difficult to continue penetration for minutes, let alone hours.
- Requires stamina in the arms and legs.
- If you give up on goals easily, this position will test your strength.
- Will cause muscular aches in the body afterward.

Press-Up Sex: Position 3

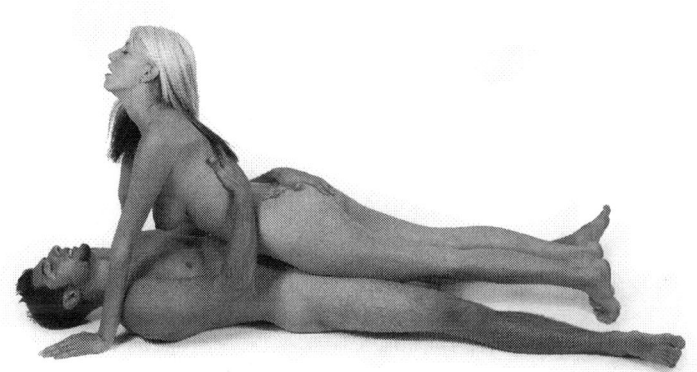

Positives:

- Gives him easy access to lick, suck, and fondle your breasts.
- This position tones the thigh and buttock muscles, if effort is applied.
- Tones the upper body and slims the abdominal area.
- Show off your "sex" face throughout lovemaking.
- Builds a deep, glowing sweat.

Negatives:

- Requires confidence, especially to show off your "orgasm" face.
- Upper body strength is necessary to remain in position.
- A general level of fitness is required to continuously thrust.
- It could cause fatigue quickly in women who do not have a sufficient level of stamina.

Press-Up Sex: Position 4

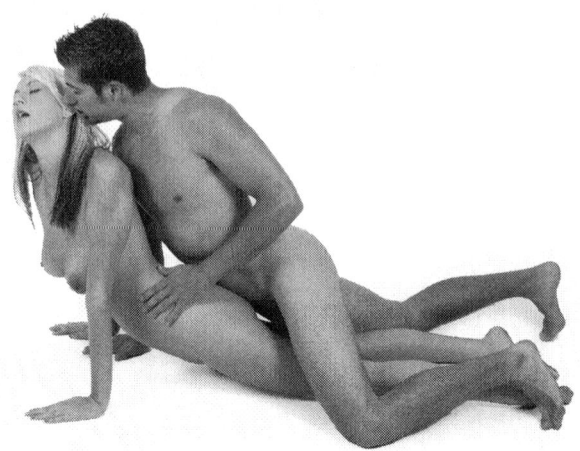

Positives:

- This position is very similar to doggy style and provides deep penetration to the female g-spot.
- The arms will tone if this position is performed consistently.
- Elongates the body and slims the abdominal area.
- He can stimulate the nape of your neck, ears, and spine with his fingers, tongue, and lips.
- Create intimacy with raunchy kisses.
- With great teamwork, this position creates a thorough toxin-cleansing sweat.
- Pain-relieving endorphins release.

Negatives:

- Requires upper body strength to carry your partner comfortably.
- Difficult to stroke the clitoris.
- Inflexible couples may find it difficult to kiss.
- Makes it difficult to view the pleasurable reactions on her face.

Upside Down Sex: Position 1

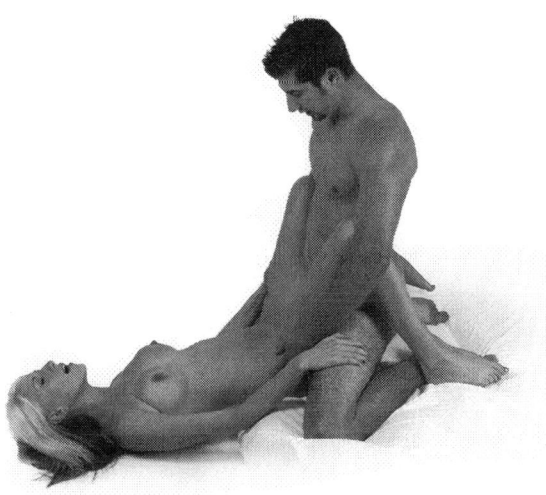

Positives:
- This position offers deep vaginal penetration.
- Display the upper half of your body with confidence, and show off your "orgasm" face during lovemaking.
- Return thrust to tone the muscles of the thigh and buttocks.
- Run your nails over his thighs to excite his senses.
- If your partner has incredible upper body strength to hold you in position, he could also stimulate your clitoris with his fingers or a toy.

Negatives:
- Difficult to embrace.
- If you hate deep penetration, this position may not be a firm favorite.
- Not ideal for shy women with body hang-ups.

Upside Down Sex: Position 2

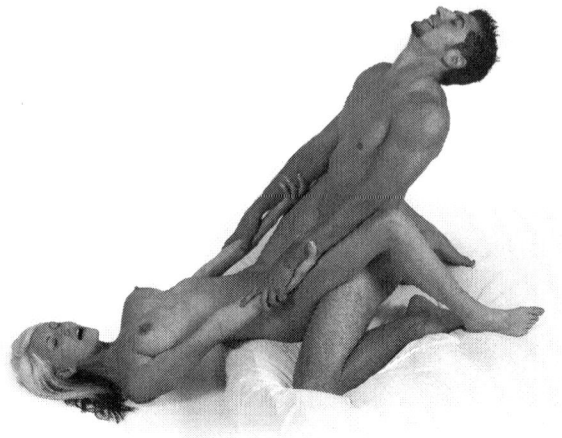

Positives:

- "Rush of blood to the head" type of sex.
- Leads to mind-blowing orgasms.
- Leaning off the bed instantly slims the abdominal area.
- Give him a great view of your bouncing breasts and "orgasm" face.
- Offers deep penetration to the g-spot, and will cause some women to turn multi-orgasmic.

Negatives:

- The positioning of sex makes it difficult for couples to embrace.
- He must have excellent upper body strength to hold you upright and stop your buttocks from slipping off the bed during sex.
- Self-confidence is paramount in order to display your body and "orgasm" face.
- If you hate deep penetration, this position may not appeal to you.

Upside Down Sex: Position 3

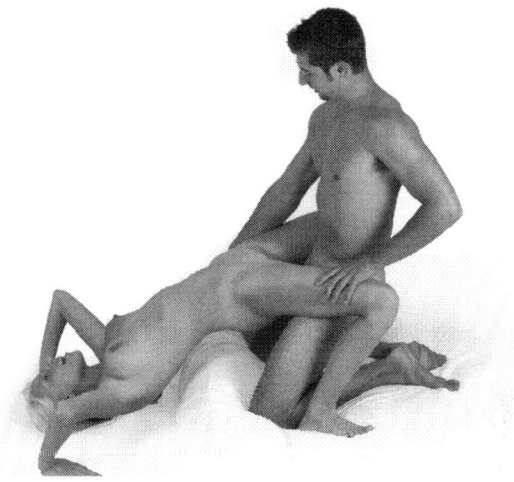

Positives:

- Tones the triceps.
- Elongates the body and slims the abdominal area.
- Provides deep vaginal penetration, while also stimulating the female g-spot.
- Give the buttocks a thorough workout with return thrusts.
- Heightens the senses.
- Your partner has easy access stroke your clitoris with his fingers or use a sex toy.

Negatives:

- This position requires upper body strength to remain in position.
- The blood rush to your head will cause a pink flush to the face and chest.
- Requires incredible stamina to return thrust.
- Bodily confidence is necessary.
- Offers no opportunity to kiss.

Upside Down Sex: Position 4

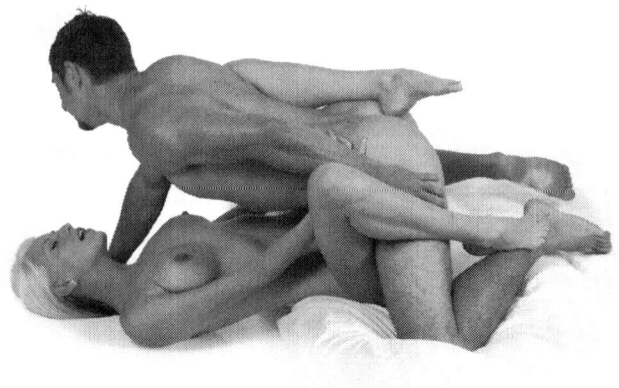

Positives:

- Give him a hot view of your beautiful breasts and facial reactions.
- Wrap your legs around him and return thrust to tone the inner thigh area and buttocks.
- Suck in the abdominals for a leaner look.
- Offers deep penetration to titillate the g-spot.

Negatives:

- Requires upper body strength from your partner in order to balance over you throughout lovemaking.
- Requires flexibility in the thigh area to wrap them around your partner comfortably.
- Flushes the face and chest.
- Requires confidence to display your body and "orgasm" face.
- Difficult to stimulate the clitoris.

Standing Sex: Position 1

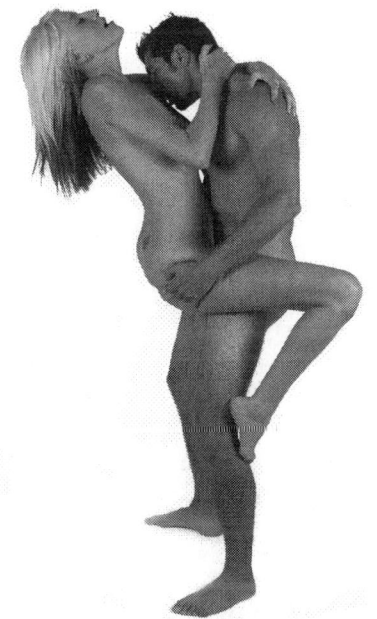

Positives:

- Builds stamina and will get you both into shape fast.
- "I can't get enough of you right now" type of sex.
- Stimulate his mind with explicit words whispered beside his ear to send shivers down his spine.
- Run your hands and nails through his hair to excite his genitals.
- Ideal "make up" sex after an argument.
- Share passionate kisses.

Negatives:

- He requires upper body strength to comfortably hold you during sex.
- Viewed as "quickie" sex, and lacks foreplay.
- Will be difficult to maintain for hours.

Standing Sex: Position 2

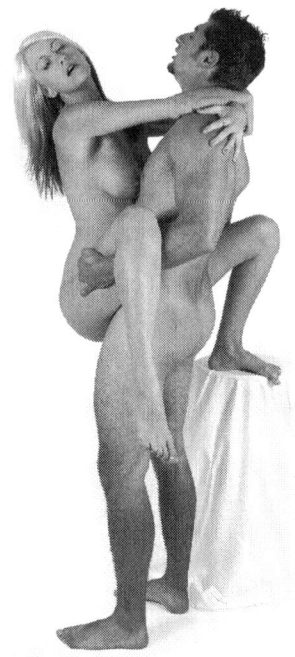

Positives:

- Rest the foot on a stool for additional support.
- Allows you both to passionately embrace.
- Use the scalp massage method to excite him further.
- Run your fingertips or nails up and down his back.
- Suck on his earlobes and whisper explicit words of excitement.

Negatives:

- Requires a good level of fitness from your partner to hold you comfortably during penetration.
- Seen as a "quickie" position.
- Does not offer the opportunity to stimulate the clitoris or participate in foreplay to build arousal before lovemaking.

Standing Sex: Position 3

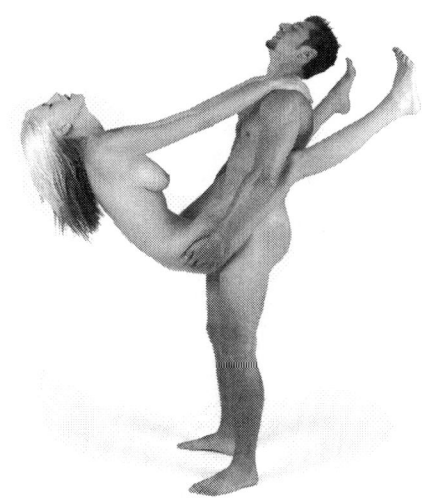

Positives:

- Give him visual satisfaction with a display of your bouncing breasts and sexually excited face.
- Gives the thigh and buttocks a great workout if you return thrust.
- Builds a detoxifying sweat.

Negatives:

- It may be difficult to return thrust, providing difficulty in toning the lower half of the body in women.
- Men require both stamina and enthusiasm to hold their partner and continuously thrust with ease.
- Difficult to kiss while you both try to retain balance.
- This position makes it difficult to stimulate the testicles or clitoris during lovemaking.

Standing Sex: Position 4

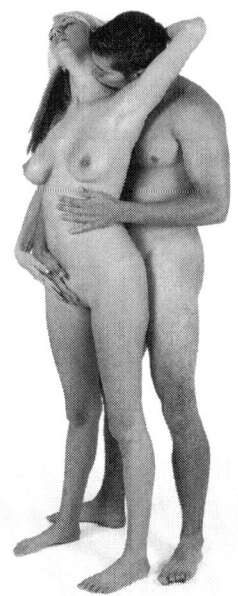

Positives:

- He can stimulate the nape of your neck and nibble your ears to send tiny shivers down the spine.
- Encourage him with a little dirty talk.
- Allow him to fondle your breasts and stroke your clitoris.
- Return thrust to tone the thigh and buttocks, and squat down slightly to cause a burn to the thighs.
- Offers deep g-spot penetration to summon vaginal orgasms.

Negatives:

- Fatigue drains the thighs, especially if your partner is tall and you have to squat down during sex.
- Women require bodily confidence, especially to tell or show him where you like to be touched.

Opposite Ends: Position 1

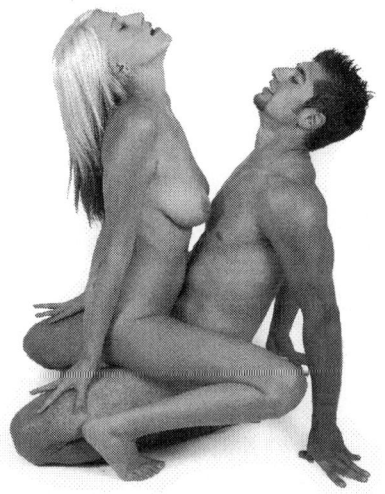

Positives:

- Excite him by rubbing your breasts against his chest.
- Easy to kiss and cuddle.
- He can stimulate your hot spots and run his fingers through your hair.
- Kiss, nibble, or whisper filthy words beside his ears to heighten his sexuality.
- The perfect position to tone the thigh and buttock muscles.
- Can thrust slower when the thighs fatigue.

Negatives:

- Requires stamina.
- Difficult to incorporate genital foreplay.

Opposite Ends: Position 2

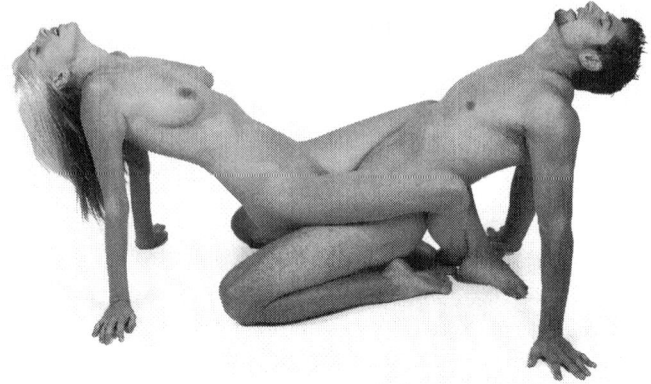

Positives:

- Displaying your body in this fashion provides visual pleasures for him during sensuous lovemaking.
- The practice of synchronized sex heightens the experience.
- Slims the abdominal area.
- Tones the thigh and buttock muscles when performed regularly.
- The triceps also get a great workout.
- If he can balance on one hand during penetration, he can use his other hand to stimulate your clitoris.

Negatives:

- Provides no opportunity to kiss.
- Requires good balance to maintain this position.
- He may be unable to reach and fondle your breasts.
- The penis may slip out several times.
- Requires a good level of stamina in both parties.
- He is unable to stimulate your erogenous zones with his lips and tongue.

Opposite Ends: Position 3

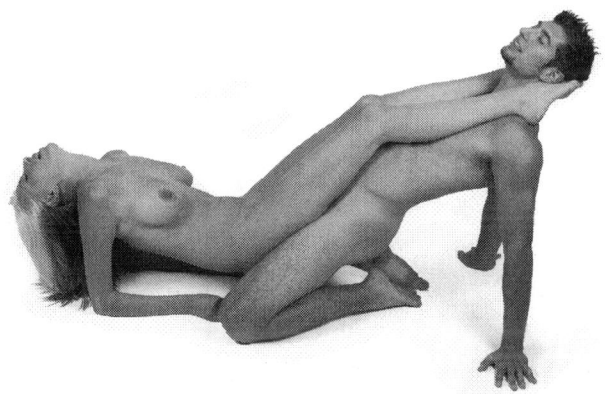

Positives:

- With effort, this position provides a full body workout, and builds a deep, detoxifying sweat.
- Give him a great view of your bouncing breasts, while his penis slips in and out of your juices.
- Elongates the body to make you appear slimmer.

Negatives:

- It may prove difficult for him to fondle your hot spots while his hands remain in position.
- Difficult to embrace.
- Requires inner thigh strength to maintain lovemaking.
- A good level of stamina is essential to continuously thrust.
- Sexual synchronicity is required to avoid his penis slipping out.

Opposite Ends: Position 4

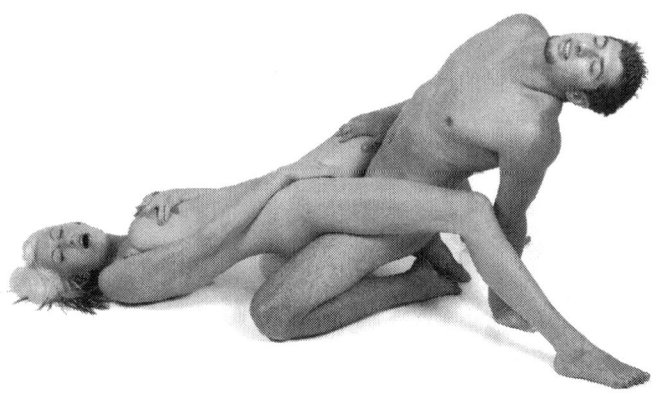

Positives:

- Provides deep thrusts to satisfy the female g-spot.
- Rub the clitoris and fondle the nipples to visually excite him.
- Enthusiastic moans will drive him crazy.
- Tones the buttock and thigh muscles if you can keep your ass upright, and meet his continuous thrusts.
- Achieve multi-orgasms through g-spot and clitoral stimulation.

Negatives:

- If this position is performed over a long period, it creates numbness in the thigh area.
- Requires stamina in the thighs and buttocks to constantly lift the pelvis and meet his every thrust.
- The penis could slip out easily without sexual rhythm.
- Self confidence is compulsory in order to visually excite him.

TIME TO GET EXPERIMENTAL

MASTURBATION

Masturbation is a healthy form of tension release. Many religions teach that you have to believe and follow what they say or else you will burn in hell, or something to that effect. People still believe this hocus-pocus. For example, having sex with the self is sinful. It is sinful only if you believe it is sinful. But why should you live in that statement and refuse yourself one of the only free pleasures of life because somebody outside of yourself stated that fact. You have free will, and right this second you can choose to think differently. I believe in God, but I do not believe in a wrathful God who will throw me into hell to be poked by a red devil. If you choose to have sex without the belief that it is a sin, your mind will be free of those manipulations.

Over the years, masturbation has been the blame as the cause of many illnesses, including asthma, epilepsy, and even mental illness. It amazes me that people believed this.

Masturbation clearly has many benefits, which is why religion works hard to make sure you do not gain this knowledge and look within. Religion equals power and mind-control. Sex relieves stress, boosts the immune system, relieves headaches, releases endorphins, and boosts the heart rate. Masturbation[48] offers the same.

With the help of your partner's touch, or use of a sex toy during masturbation, the power of your sexual mind is invoked to allow you to reach ecstasy. Experiment with solo sex and you will discover the techniques that will drop you into sexual arousal.

Unless you love sharing your sex life in the world, no one need know what you get up to in the bedroom. However, the healthy glow and enthusiasm can often give it away. Think about how you like to masturbate? Do you prefer to stroke your clitoris or penis slow or faster?

Many individuals still refrain from masturbation with the belief that it is desperate to have solo sex. Not every woman is able to achieve orgasm through penetration. Now is the time to make a change and retrain your thoughts. Step out of the guilty shell that has held you down for so long, and experience one of life's free pleasures—an orgasm.

Unless you can relax your mind and body during an intimate encounter with your partner, how can you expect to reach orgasm with him/her? Masturbation is not a desperate act—it is quite the opposite. It teaches you how to become a better lover by telling or showing your partner how you like to be touched.

Masturbation relieves tension, builds intense orgasms, and retrains the mind to enter states of multi-orgasm. Billions of individuals masturbate daily. They feel no guilt, so why should you? Use masturbation to your advantage and play sexual games with your partner through text sex, cybersex, and phone sex.

Many women find it exhilarating to allow a partner to rub her to ecstasy. It fascinates me how some individuals still abstain from solo sex and the wonderful sensation of an orgasm.

A female friend once confessed she had only ever experienced a real orgasm through masturbation, and she was thirty-five at the time. Her rabbit is between her legs satisfying her bulbous clit whenever she has a free minute available. She prefers to use a dildo rather than the fingers, but both achieve a fulfilling orgasm.

The pre-orgasmic build up is just one of the reasons why you should experiment with masturbation. If you feel confident, make a short close up video of your aroused genitals, and send it to your partner as a spontaneous surprise.

It is your choice whether to sexually experiment with masturbation. Refuse to let other people sway your decision. Follow your instincts and learn how to satisfy your body. It is my belief that masturbation is not a test of self-control throughout spiritual practice, nor will it send you straight to hell after death, if practiced regularly. I believe that the religious form of "hell" is an illusion, and if you choose to believe that hell is real, it will manifest in your life through negative situations.

I meditate almost daily and there is no way I could abstain from solo sex. I feel the sexual energy swirling around my body, which must be released, as unreleased stress is the cause of many debilitating ailments.

Every second of every day, we have amazing pleasure relieving genitals attached to our bodies. Sex is available to enjoy now, not only to conceive a child, but freely available to use as stress relief and sexual gratification.

If you want to reinstate the fireworks in your relationship, it is possible through communication and sexual experimentation with a partner. Do not turn lazy and expect that sexual chemistry will remain. True chemistry can remain in certain relationships, but rock-solid couples put in the appropriate work to ensure that desire does not wane.

Most religions still state that masturbation is a form of self-abuse and sinful. Step out of the picture and think of ways to find pleasure without sexual gratification. Okay, you can spend money on clothes, food, bills, and extravagant items, but I believe that everyone should consider free will and be willing to experience life as it should be—full of happiness, pleasure, and love. Do not let religion cloud the free pleasures of life.

Express your sexuality through masturbation, and display this to your partner. As soon as you free the power of your mind, you are back in control of your life. Orgasms are a mind-blowing form of tension release, which discharge endorphins—natural painkillers, saturating the body with warmth and satisfaction.

If you love to dabble in solo-sex, allow your partner to stroke you to ecstasy, and the finale is an emotion that will bring you closer to him/her. No face cream, however expensive, can add the glow of an orgasm to the face. Sex and orgasms are anti-aging. The more happy and joyful you feel in yourself, the less stress remains in the body, and stress is a huge degenerative ager.

Some individuals class masturbation in the same league as pornography as it is not viewed as natural. The belief is that in order to live a clean healthy life free of sin, it is important to abstain from masturbation and sexual experimentation.

It is physically impossible to immediately shed the layer of memory from the conscious mind, and I would question anyone who is able to lose the ego in a second. Everyone goes through some kind of depressive state throughout life, but your mind creates the situation, no one else is to blame. Be aware and in control, and you can change your life.

Shed Guilt And Be Aware: The Dark Night of The Soul is a stage of spiritual crisis where an individual is forced to work through repressed memories, guilt and lies. There was a point in my younger years when I believed masturbation was wrong. Who has the real evidence of this, and why should I believe them? I am a kind, generous woman letting in more light to raise my vibration.

I love sex, masturbation, and orgasms, and it is my choice to motivate this same pleasure to others. I do not wish to start a new religion, nor state I am right in what I believe, but being aware opens up the mind to so much truth.

Life should be full of light and love, not focused on fear, blame, and guilt. Sex and masturbation create a lot of repressed desire amongst the masses. In the New Age Religion, there are a lot of spiritual gurus who teach that his/her way is the only way to true happiness, but this is another manipulation of free will. Everyone has the free will to make his/her own choice. We are free to think negatively or positively, choose fear over love, or free the mind of guilt, if we choose to.

Your current reality is based on your thoughts of the past. What you think about now will shape your future. Get rid of the guilt that is perceived upon you from other people, and make your own choice about sex, masturbation, and orgasms.

Is Masturbation Good or Bad In Your View? The subconscious mind absorbs all thoughts, images, and subliminal messages like a sponge. All past memories and thoughts of guilt affect the conscious mind, unless you choose to remain aware of your thoughts, which is quite difficult to do without practice.

It is not easy to think and feel differently, but positive changes will take effect if you choose to transform your current sexual mindset through masturbation. The tension release of an orgasm can be very eye opening. Full body shivers; tears of happiness, emotional gratitude, or intense pleasures are available whenever you choose to put your focus into solo-sex. If you have never before experienced this profound pleasure, do you deny your reservations or want to awaken your sexuality within?

Orgasms are infinite. I have discovered that orgasms become stronger through frequent masturbation. Women who practice pelvic floor exercises will never have to do so ever again if the conscious choice is to masturbate regularly. After childbirth, the vagina loosens, but it can also grow slack as women age. However, regular orgasms tighten the vagina naturally and keep the area well lubricated. Kegal toning devices penetrate the vagina and the pelvic floor muscles squeeze the device, toning the vagina. Alternatively, it is possible to perform pelvic floor exercises anywhere by tensing and releasing the vaginal muscles. Neither method feels pleasant, in my view. I prefer to get a tight vagina through regular orgasms and I feel no shame. Masturbation should be praised not given the "shame game" through religious practice. During orgasm, the vaginal muscles contract sporadically, tightening the area. The body experiences warmth and pleasure during the endorphin rush when the vagina tightens and releases naturally.

There are multiple ways for a man to reach orgasm. The penis is a wonderful organ with numerous uses. Closely connected to the penis are the sensitive testicles. During arousal, the balls fill with semen before this releases during ejaculation. Men also have a male g-spot situated in the anus. During orgasm, the sphincter muscles in the anus contract, creating an incredible release of pleasure.

Men are able to ejaculate and orgasm through physical touch and mental stimulation. This is obviously dependent on the arousal provided through foreplay. Some men crave g-spot stimulation and experiment with the fingers or toys. Dependent on his open mindedness, he may share this with a partner or remain secretive and experiment alone. The sensitivity of the anus varies in men, although its diverse arousals can easily stimulate the mind. Experimentation is the only way to become familiar of the true pleasure contained within the male g-spot.

Women can reach a similar type of arousal if they are willing to push aside the stress of daily life. Insert a vibrating dildo into the vagina, and rub the clitoris with one or two fingers. During masturbation, the dual sensations work together to create an intense release, which no synthetic drug can offer naturally.

I love orgasms. During incredibly horny periods, e.g. the menstrual cycle and after the sensitivity of the first orgasm subsides, I feel ready to masturbate a second time. The extra juice secreted from my vagina often brings me to a quick climax. The second or third orgasms feel more powerful than the first, but each orgasm feels overwhelmingly different. Reaching orgasm through intercourse or masturbation relieves stress and boosts health. There is nothing harmful or sinful about masturbation.

Benefits of Masturbation

- Women can learn about the body and turn on their sexual mind through fantasy. When the clitoris is aroused, it is difficult to ignore an orgasm. Masturbation teaches a woman how to satisfy her body. Practice regularly and your orgasms will gain in power.
- Masturbation teaches a woman about her sexual preferences in order to climax during intercourse.
- It keeps the vagina moist. An unpleasant side effect of the menopause is vaginal dryness. Use the fingers or a sex toy during masturbation to further arouse the genitals. Supercharge your experience with horny fantasies. Be patient, visualize a hot scene, and continue to rub yourself until your orgasm surfaces.
- Masturbation teaches a man self-control. It is an easy form of tension release, although it can be frustrating for men who suffer from premature ejaculation. Unbelievably, regular masturbation can teach a man how to last longer during sex. Practice the squeeze technique by rubbing yourself to the brink of orgasm, before easing off slowly to prolong your

experience. Remain confident during intercourse. If you know you are performing well and satisfying your partner, you are likely to last longer.

- Practice makes perfect. During sex, prove to your partner that you know how to stimulate yourself, and give him/her a private view.

Why Masturbation Frees The Mind? My sole aim is to motivate you to free your sexual mind. Rid the mind of your subconscious guilt through Emotional Freedom Technique[49]—a form of acupuncture (without needles) where two fingers are tapped on specific acupuncture points on the body—top of head, above eyebrow, underneath eye, under nose, chin, collarbone, and under the arm, are the primary points. There is an abundance of information about Emotional Freedom Technique on the Internet. Use EFT to get rid of guilt, stress, and repressed memories. Once you feel the stress has subsided, feel even better about yourself and open up your mind to experiment with masturbation.

Break away from the illusion of controlled religion, and make your own decision about sex, orgasms, and masturbation. Society loves to manipulate the world with fear and religious bullshit; all focused to create guilt and insecurity in your mind.

I am now a better lover because I chose to walk away from the guilt and blame taught to me through Christianity. I can turn on my mind in a second if I so wish. Since the age of fourteen I have masturbated regularly, but I felt guilty for a long time. Now I am a free spirit and enjoy solo sex, whether I am in a relationship or single.

Orgasms are a natural way to relieve stress by encouraging feel good endorphins to flood the body and mind. Are we to believe that ridding the body of stress in a natural way is wrong? Conventional drugs are not the only way to relieve pain? Drugs block pain and cause the body to become immune to its own pleasurable endorphins, especially with long-term use. The body is self-healing—feed it with healthy nutrition, meditate to rid the mind of stress, and boost heart health with any form of exercise, including sex. Follow these steps and you can look forward to living a long and disease free life.

Some individuals who practice spirituality avoid sex with the belief that s/he will reach enlightenment. I use crystals, meditate, and practice various breathing techniques, including the breath of fire, taught throughout Kundalini yoga. I get sexual urges and often give in, yet I feel no guilt. Just because I choose to masturbate does not put my spiritual practice back to stage one. I do not wish to conserve sexual energy, or allow it to recycle. I would consider this to be a dangerous practice. Sexual pleasure feels divine!

Orgasm is a simple release of built up energy. However, once stress takes hold, anxiety could breed, but an orgasm frees this tension, allowing an ecstatic rush of warmth to bestow the body. Take control of your own mind; do not let the guilt of others cloud your free will.

If you want to be manipulated by religion, you could suffer from sexual inadequacies. Look at the current scandal in the Vatican and pedophilia. If religious vows cause pedophiles to emerge, is it healthy for you to follow the same? Religions also state that sex before marriage is wrong, and many individuals buy into this belief. Do not allow another person to inhibit your sexual desires. I do not state that all religions exist only to brainwash humanity, but I view it as another control of the masses. If you believe in religion, then you are not taught to think freely or to make your own choices, especially those relating to sex.

Masturbation is a natural act, but it may feel wrong to those who follow religion. I need to release my frustration through exercise, meditation, or masturbation, or I feel the growth of tension rise. I smile, enjoying the pleasure swirling through my body. Satisfaction is bliss, and we can all choose to feel that way.

Why do you care what other people think anyway? You have your own mind and body. Choose to live life however you wish. Those who judge others are envious and insecure inward. Get rid of guilt and embarrassment surrounding masturbation by becoming a patient, fulfilling lover through sexual experimentation. While other people moan about his/her unfulfilling sex life, you can smile knowing that you have the power to satisfy your body without guilt.

There are likely to be many thousands of blogs dedicated to masturbation. There is nothing arrogant about sharing your experiences with others. If it helps you to become a more experienced selfless lover, surely it's worth the effort! Hundreds of millions of individuals masturbate daily, and others less frequently. Does this knowledge now free your mind from guilt and onto sexual liberation?

If those guilty feelings do emerge, refuse to banish your newfound sexuality, but feel proud of your sexual mind. If you get a horny urge at work, nip to the toilet for a quickie. This has two instant benefits, (1) stress disappears, and (2) you can confess the steamy details to your partner afterward.

Regular masturbation has taught me how I like to be touched. I share my experiences on my blog, not to boast, but to spread the message that sex, orgasms, and masturbation manifest positive emotions. If this guide has altered your sexual thoughts and reminded you of *free will*, strip off in front of a mirror right now, and view the hot vision of your fingers stroking your genitals to a hot orgasm.

Masturbation Scenes to Trial With A Partner: Design a fun game to play with your partner and, during every sexual encounter, allow him/her to join in with your masturbating pleasure. Embrace the blissful awareness of four fingers stroking your genitals. Devise some rules of game play. An example would be to let your partner stroke your curves until you gather the confidence to perform a slow strip tease directly before masturbating.

Is it your sole aim to arouse your partner? If yes, you will surely succeed with masturbation. Continue to stroke your genitals until your partner is hard/wet and ready to explode. You will look hotter than a porno movie, and the experience will remain memorable for both parties.

- When he is totally enthralled in sports on the TV, wear a short skirt without panties for easy access. Watch how motivated he is in his sport, and stroke yourself while sat beside him. Once the heavy moans start to roll off your tongue, and he can view and hear your fingers squelching against your juices, his attention will divert away from the screen and onto your sexy body. This is a bold move and requires confidence.
- What time does your partner arrive home from work? Surprise him in your horny state by masturbating with a small clit tickler, or pounce on him and massage the balls, dovetailing his penis softly. Rub yourself to a pre-orgasmic frenzy minutes before he is due to walk through the door. On entry, he will want to compete against your fingers/toy and bring you to a fulfilling orgasm.
- Share an erotic kiss with him/her, and continue until both your bodies are pulsating with sexual desire. Play sucking games on your partner's lips and experiment with deep passionate kisses. When you cannot resist the foreplay a second longer, masturbate to synchronicity and climax together.

Can Masturbation Become Excessive? Some individuals have a higher sex drive than others. For numerous reasons, other men/women continue to feel embarrassed about masturbation and would prefer to abstain from sexual fantasies. For those who practice masturbation, however, what is excessive?

In men, excessive stimulation can over produce neurotransmitters, e.g. dopamine, serotonin, and acetylcholine and sex hormones. Excessive hormones and neurotransmitters cause the adrenal glands and brain to produce unnecessary dopamine-norepinephrine-epinephrine conversion, which cause both the body and brain functions to become extremely sympathetic. In layman terms, too much masturbation can cause physiological and psychological imbalances, e.g. weak erections, thinning hair, premature ejaculation, lower back pain, testicular pain and eye floaters.

Expert's state that ejaculation should not be performed more than two to three times per week, although I believe that solo-sex once a day is fine. However, men who practice the squeeze technique are able to orgasm without ejaculation, and this is a healthy practice.

Over masturbation can cause problems with concentration and memory, a side effect of the brain being drained of acetylcholine. Too much masturbation therefore drains important hormones and nutrients.[50]

In women, excessive masturbation can exhaust the adrenal response, which overproduces the inflammatory hormones, resulting in pain. If collagen scar tissue is formed before the clitoral and g-spot nerves are damaged, you will experience numbness in the area. Sexual desire is likely to persist, until the pituitary gland produces enough prolactin to prevent arousal.

During sexual activity and before the release of estrogen, the sex organs and adrenal glands produce androgen. The hypothalamus releases dopamine, which creates sexual arousal. During excitement to the genitals, the neurotransmitter, acetylcholine is released into the bloodstream of the sex organs. The enzyme, nitric oxide synthase, produced from the endothelium in the blood vessels, produces the gas nitric oxide. This then triggers another neurotransmitter, cyclic GMP. On its command, the blood vessels relax and increase blood flow to the sex organs. Engorgement of the genitals puts pressure on the veins, and as arousal increases, the neurotransmitter, GABA releases, increasing dopamine levels and ignites the feeling of euphoria felt during an orgasm.

After sexual activity, the enzyme PDE5 disables cyclic GMP, and the production of nitric oxide decreases, causing the sex organs to stabilize. Prostaglandin E-1 is released to relax the muscle and tissue fibers. Finally, the pituitary gland releases oxytocin—producing a feeling of satisfaction after sex and orgasm—and also prolactin, which reduce the levels of testosterone in men and estrogen in women. Serotonin is also released to modulate sexual desire.

These processes can go into overdrive and stress out the body if you over exert yourself through excessive sexual activities. Excess dopamine overproduces epinephrine, which pushes the body into a continuous state of fight-or-flight. If you consider that your body has to undergo this process *every* time you orgasm, it is extremely taxing on the body.[51]

As long as you're not masturbating five or six times a day, solo-sex is a healthy practice. I often masturbate once or twice a day dependent on how horny I feel, and suffer no complications. Some women are especially horny during the menstrual period and may experience stronger than usual orgasms.

Happily married couples or those in long-term relationships still indulge in masturbation. There is nothing wrong or dishonest about masturbating in private. Achieving orgasm releases tension, and a huge majority of people worldwide masturbate at all times of the day. If they feel no shame, why should you?[52]

Hot Masturbation Tips For Women

- Close the eyes and imagine a hot fantasy starring your partner. Alternatively, visualize stepping into a secret fantasy, or experiment with your favorite fetish. Do you have a major crush on a celebrity and feel too embarrassed to admit this to your partner? As a heterosexual woman, do you ever imagine how it would feel to pleasure another female orally? The fantasy could be mild or wildly explicit. Make it different and allow your sexual mind to live out its potential.

- Experiment with masturbation in various locations. Have text, phone, or cybersex with your partner at work. If there are colleagues hovering nearby, allow your partner to arouse you until you have to rush to the bathroom for relief. After your orgasm, write down your explicit thoughts and feelings, and read the story to him/her in the evening.

- With a fantasy firmly fixed in your mind, think about how you would react if it were to become a reality. Would you become a horny minx or turn shy? What are your exact thoughts and fantasies? Does your body feel sexual? Is your throat dry because your vagina has stolen all your juices? If you are normally shy and reserved, do you ever wonder how it would feel to become the girl of your partner's dreams? You *can* become whoever you wish to be through the power of thought. Tell yourself you are sexy and powerful, and you will become exactly that person.

- Free your anxiety through meditation. When the mind is free of tension, your sexual mind is open and free to visualize horny thoughts. Stroke your skin with your fingertips or nails, excite the nipples, caress and cup the breasts, and focus on your orgasmic fulfillment.

- Brush a finger between your thighs, and saturate your fingers with your pheromone-enriched juices. Stroke the inside of your thigh and brush one or two fingers over the labia. When you feel ready to masturbate, stroke your anatomy, while enjoying every guilt-free sensation. Do you throb with desire for an orgasm, or do you ache for sexual penetration? If you prefer to use a toy, there are lots to choose from, many of which will cause a sudden orgasmic release.

- Fingers and toys stimulate the genitals. The inside of the thigh is a highly sensitive area to caress in both men/women. Stimulate this area during foreplay.

- Rub the clitoris with one or two fingers, or keep the middle finger on the clitoris and use the ring and index finger to stroke the outer vaginal lips. It feels horny to keep the clitoris wet with juices. Stroke yourself slowly to drive your mind and body alert for orgasmic release.

- Keep all sexual thoughts at the forefront of your mind, and experiment with varied finger pressures. When you feel close to the peak, slip your fingers away from your clit, and finger yourself to stimulate the female g-spot. This could create an urge to urinate and generate a squirting orgasm.

- Quickie orgasms are effective, but long masturbation sessions create rapid heart rate, perspiration, and an intense build up of sexual emotions. Masturbation is a great workout if you put forth the effort and time. An increase in heart rate expels toxins and gives the skin a healthy glow from within. Warming endorphins saturate the body with pleasure, and when the body heat rises through exercise, e.g. masturbation and sex, calories burn through the increase in the metabolic rate.

- Experiment with varied rubbing techniques. Circle your clitoris with two fingers, or rub your clitoris in a figure of eight. Both methods work to create diverse sensations. Although it could take longer to climax with these methods, it's worth the wait.

- Use your sexual mind to focus on a hot fantasy, while your fingers stroke your clitoris to an explosive climax. The clitoris grows full and fat and throbs for attention. Pull back your clitoral hood with your other hand, if it feels more pleasurable. Do not hold the breath during climax. It is hard enough to relax during daily life, so practice deep breaths to help your body remain free of tension. Once you know how to relax your breaths, it becomes easier to transfer this technique into lovemaking with your partner.

- Allow sensual imagery to create an orgasmic build up. Continue to fantasize, stroke the clitoris, and synchronize your mind and body to build a wonderful orgasm.
- After explosion, let the warm endorphins rush through your entire body. The clitoris is always sensitive to touch afterward, but this settles after just ten to fifteen minutes.
- Masturbation is an easy form of stress release. Imagine how it will feel to experience an orgasm during lovemaking with your partner. Do you think it will delight him to watch you masturbate? Show your partner how you like to be touched. Do you enjoy fast or slow strokes, g-spot penetration with fingers or a toy, or varied circling pressures on the clit? The sound of your juices rubbing across your clitoris will turn on your partner, who will now be eager to pleasure you in every possible way.

Hot Masturbation Tips For Men
- Firstly, do not feel guilty or uptight about masturbation. It is perfectly natural and supposed to be fun. It's time to relax and enjoy yourself.
- Focus on a location where you can relax and not fret about any interruptions that could alarm you.
- Follow your sexual instincts and listen to your bodily reactions. Stand in front of a mirror and imagine that your partner or celebrity crush is pleasuring you in exactly the same way you love to masturbate. Imagine the cock now stood firmly in your hand is sliding in and out of your partner's mouth.
- Experiment with different techniques, speeds, pressures, and locations.
  - Standard: Pump with closed thumb and fingers wrapped around the penis.
  - Form an imitation vagina by interlocking your fingers; then close them around your penis.
  - Rub your penis between the palms and fingers, much like you would when rubbing a stick to start a fire.
  - Use the standard pump technique, but use two hands. Add a twisting motion from each hand to vary the sensation.

- o Tap the penis against your abdomen, or flick your head up and down over a smooth surface or counter edge to produce a strong hardness.
- Try varied positions. Lie with your legs spread, knees pulled up, or raise the legs. Try standing in front of a mirror. Squat slightly, spread the legs, and masturbate until you climax. Be creative.
- Try various locations e.g. the bedroom, shower, and/or the outdoors. Be risqué, but make sure that it is a safe location. Outdoors on a deck or patio after dusk can be a turn on.
- Set a date, time, and place, and let yourself go. Have no fear about moaning, shaking your ass, or writhing to the marvelous sensations occurring from the sexual imagery stirring through your mind.
- When you feel your orgasm building to a peak, grip the base of your shaft, rub harder until your legs turn to jelly and you no longer feel in control, and squirt semen onto your fingers.
- If you prefer to send out powerful long jets of semen, squeeze the pelvic floor muscles before each squirt. However, watch out for the eyes!
- Prolong the experience. Do not rush your climax. Tease yourself until your balls feel heavily loaded, and then continue to keep yourself on the edge with quick firm strokes. Slow down the strokes to lengthen your orgasmic release.
- If visual excitement stirs your mind into arousal, glance at a couple of filthy websites, or browse through an explicit book/magazine. Men are visual, and any hint of female flesh could provoke an instant reaction between his legs. Whether you are single or coupled, imagine a hot fantasy starring just your partner. Is it a threesome fantasy you image or perhaps a lesbian romp? Do not put your only focus on magazines or porno movies, but use the power of your mind to visualize a hotter fantasy.
- When your dick is excited, add lotion or oil—optional but horny—and rub it into steel. Play out the hot fantasy until you climax.
- Do you love tugging on your balls, or do you prefer to massage them softly? Some men find that their testicles become extra sensitive during arousal, but other men prefer a harder tug.
- If you are open to experimentation, widen your legs and gently rim the ass with a finger or soft jelly toy until you feel the urge to experiment a little deeper. This will feel extremely erotic for most men. After the

- rimming stage, massage the g-spot (found two inches inside the anus), until you reach climax.
- Would you like to experience multiple sensations? Stimulate the g-spot, penis, and testicles at the sane time. Your partner may need to help you out with this scene, but I am confident that you will reach new depths of pleasure.
- Build up a steady friction during masturbation and, before explosion, back off with gentle rubbing for a couple of minutes. View your fingers as the weapon of power, and release your orgasm when the sensations feel overwhelming.
- Dependent on your arousal, pre-cum could dribble from the tip of your penis. Rub this into your dick, and increase/decrease the friction of your strokes. Slow teasing heightens the sensations, plus it also keeps the penis rock hard and alert for more stimulation.
- Moan heavily and let your body writhe. Feel the sexual tension build in your genitals, and go with the original image you first visualized, which pushed you into this horny stage.

If you have decided that you and your partner are ready to experiment with sex, you now need to develop the self-confidence necessary to mutually masturbate with your partner. Stroke your genitals until you climax over your partner's face or another favorite part of her anatomy. This can be fun…but also annoying, especially if she dislikes semen squirted on her face or body.

Masturbation is also a fun tool to use in any sexual scene; it improves orgasms, turns individuals multi-orgasmic, and can help you become a more satisfying lover.

During orgasm, men release a sleep hormone, which could make it difficult for him to remain awake. If this is you, try to cuddle your partner to make her feel important. After orgasm, women release oxytocin, a hormone that builds intimacy. This is the reason why women often become hooked on men soon after lovemaking. Women are not designed to have no strings sex.

Hot Masturbation Tips For Couples

- Masturbate in alternative surroundings, perhaps while driving, during a walk in the erotic rain, or on the beach during vacation. A very simple but appealing scene is to view your naked body in front of a mirror. The latter can feel incredibly liberating for women especially, as many are critical of themselves. Women view lumps and bumps that a partner may never notice. The negative subconscious mind mocks her as unworthy, however, stating positive affirmations can alter this, e.g. "My body is sexy and gorgeous," or "I love every inch of my body." For best results, repeat them fifty to one hundred times daily in front of a mirror.

- Surrender to your partner's fingers and tongue during domination foreplay. Remember to relax in the moment to build an intense orgasm.

- Be spontaneous; yet remain secretive about the sexual thoughts fizzing through your mind. Dominate your partner in the middle of the night, or use your tongue and fingers to seduce his dick, until he groans your name. Force him to grip your hair before you release his climax.

- If you prefer to masturbate in private, take a deep confident breath and give your partner a show s/he will never forget. Most individuals are taught to think negatively regarding sex, and if any feelings of guilt become evident, share the issue(s) with your partner. The deeper you practice a sexual art, including masturbation, the more natural it comes, and the less of an emotional burden it holds over you.

- Rub your genitals over your partner's, until you both explode with sexual ecstasy.

- I realize this is a little naughty, but it's often necessary. Phone work and explain that your stomach feels dodgy after last night's dinner. Lower your tone of voice to sound convincing. If you are an honest and hardworking individual, remember that everyone is entitled to a sick day. Forget what it costs the taxpayer. It's time you claimed a reward for what you put into the monetary system. Let go of guilt, and remind yourself of the fun you will experience with your partner.

- Experiment with a fun foreplay method you have never before tried with your partner. Perhaps you have both decided to tryout anal sex. Spend all day on foreplay, heavily lubricate the area, then experiment when you both feel ready.

Admire Yourself In Front of a Mirror: There is nothing pretentious about admiring the true beauty that is you. See it as a positive step to enlighten your self-image. Before stripping off your clothes, take a few minutes to gather your thoughts. Repeat positive affirmations—state them with determination and feeling. Tell yourself you are sexy and desirable, and **believe** it. What does your partner love about you? Bring up those compliments and turn them into positive affirmations. Banish your internal critic.

Do you notice your best assets, e.g. a tiny waist, hourglass figure, come to bed eyes laced with eyeliner, supple squeezable breasts, or hair free soft skin. However you feel about yourself inward, your partner already loves every inch of you. A positive affirmation to state every day is "I love and accept myself just the way I am."

Learn to love your body today. State the affirmation while you are stood in front of a mirror. Nobody is perfect inside and out. The world hopes to present perfection through beauty products, hair salons, and healthy foods, but you can make a wise choice to love yourself right now and stop looking outside of your self for happiness.

Supermodels and celebrities are paid huge amounts of money to maintain the "perfect" figure, but it is not a healthy practice to chain smoke, drink bottled water, and eat a couple of apples per day. The media hype about body shape and diet is more than a little gloomy, would you agree? Once you make the choice to step out of your critical shell, and embrace the body that Mother Nature blessed you with, your self-confidence will shine through.

I will always have a bit of fat on my booty and thighs, but who cares! I refuse to diet. My heart is healthy, and I enjoy exercise, especially spinning, boxing, and weight training. I practice various breathing techniques, which pump my body with fresh oxygen. Be thankful for your health, and show off your figure with confidence. Believe in yourself and your positive self-talk will eventually transfer to your subconscious mind, thus affecting your current mindset and reality.

This next move requires confidence, but if you continue to re-affirm positive statements, your self-confidence will improve dramatically.

- Strip off your clothes and admire your body in front of the mirror. This is what your partner sees and loves, so start believing in yourself.
- For women, caress your curves, beautiful breasts, and smile at your naked reflection without allowing it to inflate your ego. For men, admire your biceps, strong thighs, and masculinity.
- Close the eyes and visualize a hot fantasy. Alternatively, if your imagination lacks inspiration, read erotic literature. Imagine your partner is stroking you exactly where you stand or lie, but view it through the mirror so it appears real.

- Use your fingertips to stimulate the skin, or use a feather or piece of silky material to titillate the body. Close your eyes and feel every delightful sensation. Omitting a sense works to heighten others.

- Embrace the sight of your fingertips caressing your breasts, massaging your inner thighs, and exciting your clitoris. Pull back the clitoral hood and view the plumpness of your clitoris, as you focus on the pleasure churning through your mind. Use sexy thoughts to reach incredible heights of ecstasy.

- Rub oil or pre-cum into the tip of your penis, and then massage the shaft to turn it from semi-hard to granite. Continue to brush your fingers over the shaft until you feel ready to pull harder. This technique builds stronger orgasms, plus it could also help you to last longer during sex.

- Do you prefer to masturbate alone, or will you allow your partner to stroke you to ecstasy. Arousal will heighten during this stage. If you are alone in the room, imagine your partner is there with you watching you masturbate. This should send pleasurable tingles down your spine.

- Observe the flirty thoughts flowing through your mind, and notice how your genitals grow in arousal through the mirror. Are your nipples hard and excited? Do your knees quiver before climax? Is your face expressive during orgasm? Both men/women love to watch the pleasure on a partner's face during penetration and orgasm.

- Would you prefer your partner to stroke you to ecstasy? If yes, give your partner feedback with deep fervent moans and writhe. Whisper words of encouragement beside his/her ear to further stimulate his/her senses.

- Stroke the genitals simultaneously. Four hands stimulating the genitals is an amazing experience to remember. Furthermore, confessing of the pleasure you feel displays self-assurance.

- During masturbation, do you circle your clitoris with your finger or a toy? How does it feel to be in control of your orgasm? Do you feel exhilarated? Build up the sensation until you feel the urge to let yourself go. Remain aware of your bodily reactions until you climax.

- Use sex toys to vary the sensations of masturbation. Men can tickle the testicles or the tip of the penis with a vibrating egg—you may find one of these in your partner's goody drawer. This excites the genitals in multiple ways. Give your partner free reign to pleasure your genitals until you climax.

- With the knowledge of how you like to touch yourself during masturbation, does it feel easier to play in front of your partner? If you feel over confident, record a short movie on your phone, and send him/her the video of your naughty exploits.
- Viewing your partner licking, caressing, and rubbing his/her fingers against your naked body and genitals unleashes an abundance of sexual desire.
- Talk explicitly to your partner, e.g. "Do you want my lips wrapped around your dick," or "Do you want me to rub my cock over your juicy clit?" Both are expressive and sexual. Turn the conversation exciting, memorable, and hot enough to turn your partner rampant with sexual desire for you.

Does it feel liberating to watch your body orgasm through the mirror, or does it excite you to actively participate in mutual masturbation? Persevere with solo-sex until it feels second nature. The guilty beliefs will soon vanish from your ego.

Share all of your likes/dislikes with your partner. This helps to create intimacy and builds a close bond where you are able to orgasm together. Great sex requires mental release and relaxation. Tension creates anxiety, which can affect sexual performance.

Rid the mind of worries with deep breaths. If you still struggle to banish the guilt, take a deep breath and minimize all those negative, disempowering thoughts by visualizing the images disappearing to the left mental screen of your consciousness. Practice this skill regularly, and soon enough your sexuality will shine through, and guilt-free masturbation will feel like second nature.

ORAL SEX

Oral sex is a very intimate act between couples, as it requires confidence, trust, and relaxation, especially if you plan to offer the most intimate part of your body to be pleasured. Oral sex is best performed when the body is clean, relaxed, and alert for attention.

Always bathe beforehand so that your partner cannot complain. It is possible to alter the taste of your sexual juices by eating plenty of alkaline foods e.g. fruits and vegetables. Men are able to alter their semen easily through the diet, but it can take weeks or months to alter the taste of seminal fluids in women. Nobody wants to pleasure unsightly scented genitals, so it is important to bathe or shower daily. Alternatively, use baby wipes to cleanse the genital area.

Uncircumcised men must focus on washing the internal and external areas of the foreskin thoroughly. In women, the vaginal lips should be cleansed with a PH wash, preferably non-scented. Clean only the external area of the vagina, never the internal, as the vagina is naturally self-cleansing to prevent bacteria or thrush.

If the thought of oral sex creates a stirring panic, experiment in the shower when your partner's genitals are pristinely clean. Oral sex in the bath could prove difficult, unless the tub is spacious. Shared Jacuzzi's are unhygienic and are best avoided. Avoid intercourse or giving/receiving oral sex in a Jacuzzi.

Sexual Juices: Every individual has his/her own unique sexual scent, which is secreted through the genitals. Pre-cum secretes from the penis before an orgasm, and women dribble juices from the vagina during arousal. The taste of these juices could vary from musky to sweet and unique.

If you have never felt the confidence to experience your own flavor, why don't you experiment now? It will not kill you, nor do I doubt it will taste as foul as turnip juice. Has your partner given you feedback of how you tasted unique and sweet? This is positive.

Most individuals grow paranoid about the scent of his/her genitals and the taste of seminal fluids. However, if your diet is full of fresh fruit and vegetables, you should have a very unique and pleasant flavor.

Cunnilingus Tips For Men: Use the fingers, tongue, and lips to stimulate her clitoris. Experiment with various moves, e.g. listen for moans, recognize her writhing body, and remain confident in your abilities of hitting her hot spots.

Ensure that your partner is relaxed and ready for your moves. Not every woman is able to relax and enjoy this very intimate foreplay. The natural odor from the genitals could create her paranoia and anxiety. However, most men feel overpowered and horny when faced with the scent of a woman. The mere touch of a wet vagina, or the view of an ecstatic face is often more than enough to arouse a man. If she feels tense during oral sex, relax her beforehand with a shoulder or scalp massage.

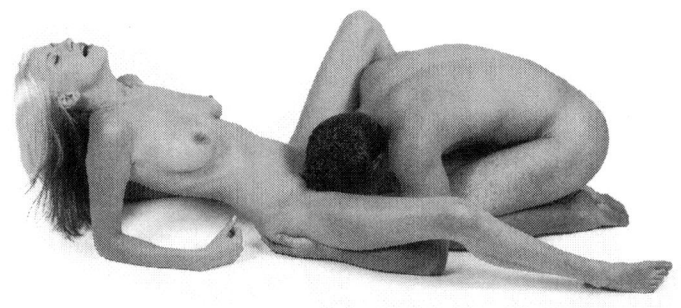

- **Vary Your Technique**: Think about how you will stimulate your partner's genitals. Will you use your fingers, tongue, or a sex toy? If you feel confident and want to bring her to a memorable orgasm, why not use all three?
- **Take Your Time**: Performing oral sex on a partner requires patience and great self-control. Cunnilingus should never be rushed. Beads of sweat form in the vagina during arousal creating the lush wetness. However, even though she is feeling sexual, her pleasure should not be rushed...EVER. Be a considerate and patient lover and her orgasm will reward your efforts.
- **Tease**: Caress her inner thigh with your fingers and tongue. Make her beg for oral pleasure. Creating desire in a woman is a courageous move.

Vary your stimulations to excite her body and mind. If you are able to relax her mind, she can then surrender to the bliss on offer from your "pleasuring" tools.

- **Clitoral Hood**: The protective hood surrounds the sensitive clit. When aroused, the clitoris darkens, grows in size, and starts to poke out from under the hood. Pull back the hood gently to further excite your partner.

- **Suck The Clitoris**: Masturbation feels ecstatic for many women, but during oral sex, her true emotions will surface. Surprising her with the gift of cunnilingus has two benefits: (1) it creates trust, depths of passion, and orgasmic pleasure to build in her, and (2) it rests your hardworking tongue.

- **Enquire**: Does she masturbate? If yes, she knows exactly what depth of touch and penetration is required to reach orgasm. If you can relax her mind and body with a massage beforehand, she may be more likely to confess this personal information. Not every woman enjoys finger penetration or a dildo fuck. Enquire with her as to what she likes/dislikes. A wet vagina does not indicate that she desires finger penetration or hard sex. Be polite and respectful of her needs. The female g-spot is situated in the vagina. Once stimulated, this hot spot produces a translucent veil of lubrication. Make her beg for more by creating impatience in her hot spots.

- **Keep The Clitoris Moist**: Drive her into a manic frenzy by applying lots of moisture to her clit. Use saliva, pre-cum, oil, food, or bottled lubricants to keep her on edge.

- **Rimming**: Does she enjoy finger penetration during oral sex? Does she enjoy her ass rimmed by your tongue? The sensitive anus is a hot erogenous zone to stimulate in both men/women. If she's a little reluctant at first, build up her orgasm by stroking her clit, and then experiment on her ass.

- **Vary Your Technique**: Lick across the clit, side to side, and up and down. Alternatively, circle the clit with the fingers and tongue. Drive her crazy by rubbing the inside of her thighs with every stroke of her clit.

- **Dominate**: The sight of your partner naked is hot enough, but if you want a powerful reaction from her, use the power of domination to control her pleasure. Ask her to lift her buttocks, squeeze her flesh, and then sink your head between her legs. Use your titillating tongue to make her wriggle further and fuck your face.

- **Excite Her G-Spot**: The female g-spot is situated approximately two inches inside the vaginal wall. It feels fleshy on first contact and can create a variety of sensations in women. Doggy style is one position that offers deep penetration, but finger penetration can also create diverse pleasures. Toys are perfect to use on the g-spot. Cause her multi-orgasmic pleasure with simultaneous vaginal and clitoral excitement. Set yourself a tough challenge, but follow it through with exciting foreplay. Give her no excuse to fake an orgasm.

- **Invite Her To Play The Game**: Foreplay is designed to enhance your partner's pleasure to help her achieve orgasm. If you are able to bring her to orgasmic fulfillment, she will view you as a sex God. Request that she joins in the game. While stroking her g-spot and clitoris, ask her to masturbate. If is often difficult for a man to focus on every aspect of the female anatomy, and it could even cause anxiety in some shy men. Watching her masturbate will excite you in multiple ways, while also creating an intimate connection between you both.

- **Make Eye Contact**: During oral sex, maintain strong eye contact with your partner. This helps to create desire and will extend her levels of trust and confidence in your abilities.

- **Avoid The Clitoris**: I love to masturbate in this way. When my lover is stroking me and teasing my outer vaginal lips and labia, deliberately avoiding my clitoris drives me nuts! Stimulate the area around the clitoris, and when she becomes juicy, avoid the clitoris to build a fervent desire that she will struggle to hide. Make her beg for her orgasmic release.

Fellatio Tips For Women: A large number of men enjoy blowjobs occasionally or very frequently. If you display enthusiasm during oral sex why should he look elsewhere for the same pleasure? You will remain a memorable sex Goddess through his eyes.

- **Show Enthusiasm**: Men love to watch their partner giving oral sex, but what they love especially are enthusiastic efforts. If you resist or pull a sulky face during oral sex, it could discourage his pleasure. Men are able to instinctively notice the resistance in women, which could affect him sexually. Stay optimistic with firm eye contact throughout.

- **Make Eye Contact**: Give him the "come to bed" eyes during oral sex, then wink at him before sucking him harder or faster. A display of intense eye contact shows him how much you love the intimate act.

- **Tease**: The inner thigh is a sensitive area to titillate in both men/women. Use the fingers; tongue, and/or vibrating toys to further build his levels of sexual desire. When he starts to thrash wildly, dominate his shaft with deep firm sucks, and masturbate him with firm strokes into your mouth.

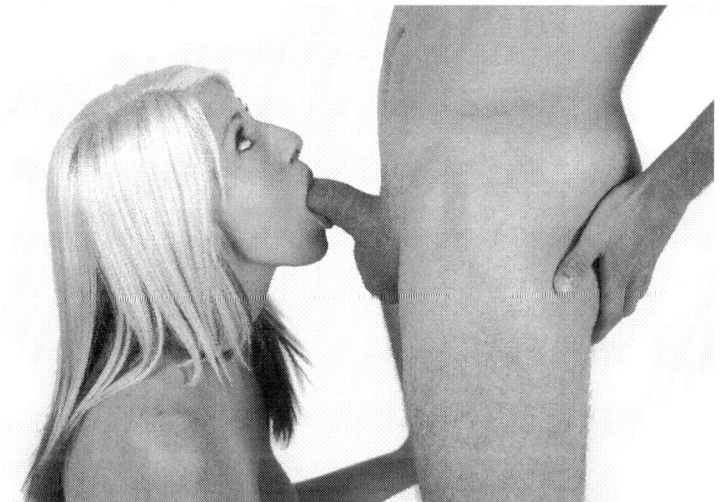

- **Tender Testicles**: During arousal, the testicles fill with semen creating heaviness and heightened sensitivity. Be careful not to harm this area during oral pleasure. Some men prefer the testicles to be massaged softly, rather than sucked. Listen for his feedback and watch his expressive face to find out his likes/dislikes. Alternatively, ask him how he likes to be touched. This is always a winning combination.

- **Use Your Tongue**: Grip the base of his penis before allowing his tip to enter your mouth. Minutes before he is due to experience the delight of your lips surrounding his dick, tease your tongue around his tip hardening him further, and force his dick to find its way into your mouth. By this stage, it will be hard, full, and ready to fire.

- **Moisturize**: If your mouth does not drool with saliva during oral sex, you may not be putting forth vigorous effort. Fellatio is supposed to be messy, but it also gives your partner extreme pleasure and the view of your enthusiasm. Real oral sex will look nothing like a celebrity cloned sex video. Rub excess saliva into his balls and shaft to build up his orgasm.

When his tip has dribbled enough pre-cum, mix it with your saliva, and keep him on edge with long deep sucks. Excite his penis with a variety of slow and soft teasing, then alternate deep sucks to give him an out of this world orgasmic experience.

- **Use Fingers and Toys**: Deep rubs are often preferred against soft finger strokes over the penis and testicles, especially during masturbation. If you can read his feedback, you should know when he's at his peak. Slow down the strokes when he's almost ready to fire. The gentle brush of your fingers over his shaft will keep him begging for more. Massage the dick tenderly and create suction around the tip of his penis to blow his mind. Each time you rub his shaft, allow him to fuck your mouth gently, but continue to suck him vigorously.

- **Build The Pressure**: Each time his dick enters your mouth, suck the tip harder and rub his slippery shaft (full of pre-cum and saliva) with both hands to create a deep friction. Is he normally shy to make the first move? If so, I hope the oral pleasure you give him will cause deep implausible moans to roll off his tongue. If he shakes and pre-cum squirts from his tip before ejaculation and orgasm—even better.

- **Fondle The Male G-Spot**: This hot spot is situated one to two inches inside the anus and is potent enough to turn some men multi-orgasmic. If the idea of arousing this area fills you with dread or embarrassment, consider his pleasure. After a bath or shower, rim his anus with a soft jelly toy, or use a combination of your fingers and tongue to build up his excitement. Foreplay is often instinctive so you will be able to decipher if he is enjoying your move by noticing his body language. Stimulating the male g-spot could cause pre-ejaculation to seep from his tip, but it can also turn most men multi-orgasmic.

- **Control The Depth**: This is dependent on his penis size, but if he is above average, you must consider your comfort during oral sex. If you push his penis into your mouth far too deeply, gagging, streaming eyes, or even vomiting could surface. Use the hands to control his depth of penetration, and continue to seduce him with intense eye contact, and use your magic tongue and fingers to bring him to a powerful release.

- **Deep Throating**: I love giving head, but I hate deep throating. Men can create visual delight by viewing this on porno movies. However, performing this deed in reality can induce vomiting, especially if you are unable to control his penis size during oral sex. Driving a man to incredible heights of ecstasy during oral sex does not require deep throating or award winning tricks. Use your seductive tongue, soft fingers, and a selection of sex toys to create a memorable experience. Less is often more when giving oral pleasure to a man.

- **Teeth Caution**: Oral sex is an act largely based on trust, so be careful that your teeth do not get in the way during fellatio. This can happen if your concentration falters. Oral sex is a skill. If you experiment regularly, you will build up a good technique. One second of discomfort from the teeth could cause his erection to fade, so be careful, especially if you're into deep throating. In my experience, I have found that brushing the teeth very lightly over the penis can also heighten his pleasure. Listen for pleasurable moans or look for positive feedback in his body language.
- **Swallow Occasionally**: During oral sex and after orgasm, men like to view their partner swallowing semen. Male ejaculation is healthy and a great source of zinc and protein. Semen should contain no aftertaste, but if there is an unpleasant flavor, simple changes in the diet can alter his flavor. Do not feel under pressure to swallow; experiment only when you feel ready.

The 69er:[53] I have never been a fan of the 69er position. However, it is a very pleasurable position for many couples. Personally, I find that it distracts my mind from fulfilling its mission—to bring my partner to a hot orgasm. I prefer to focus one hundred percent concentration on my partner during oral sex. Sit on your partner's face, or allow him to sit on yours.

After experimenting with this position in the past, I found it easier to sit on my partner's face and focus on his oral pleasure, but then I struggled to relax in the moment and reach my own fulfilling orgasm. Sitting on a man's face requires confidence, but he'll love the view. If you find it difficult to concentrate *and* orgasm during the 69er, focus your energies on one-on-one oral loving.

Who should take the initiative with oral sex you may wonder? If you feel confident, take charge of your partner after a stressful day at work, or design a fun text messaging game to entice your partner to crave every inch of your body. Flip a coin, ask difficult questions that you know s/he will struggle to answer, or make up another rule. The list is endless.

ANAL SEX

Anal sex is often a tricky subject for most couples to discuss. Anal sex is still viewed as high risk and an area never to experiment with during foreplay, but other individuals find it to be a highly erotic zone that deserves much attention and pleasure.

Whether you are for or against the idea of anal sex, it is important to note that this area is full of sensitive nerve endings that affect the male/female genitals on stimulation. The penis, fingers, anal beads, vibrating toys, tongue, and dildos are individual fun ways to excite the anus and cause men/women to reach multi-orgasmic states.

In men, the anus is one of the hottest erogenous zones in the body because the g-spot resides two inches inside the anal wall. When both homosexual and heterosexual couples open up the mind and experiment with this area, new phases of sexual excitement are felt in the body and mind.

The male g-spot is often stimulated during orgasm in highly sensitive men. Other men remain curious about the anus, but refrain from titillating this hot spot, until one day they experience the potency of the g-spot during sex, orgasm, or masturbation.

It is important to communicate with your partner. Confess of your likes/dislikes in the bedroom, including your desires, adventurous sexual fantasies, and fetishes. If you are shy about expressing a kinky side, how will your partner learn of your cravings?

Do you continue to believe that anal sex is disgusting? If so, those exact thoughts may influence your partner to think in the same way. The mind is extremely powerful and gives you want you desire. It is forever processing your thoughts and visualizations. Instead of focusing on the desire you DO NOT want, start to focus on those you DO want. Would it surprise you to know that many women love anal sex, and a high degree of women are open to experimentation?

It is easy to venture into experimental phases of sex without communicating your desire to a partner. Bathe and clean the area beforehand, and then lubricate your finger or squirt KY jelly onto a sex toy, e.g. anal beads or a dildo. You may feel a couple of seconds of discomfort, but everyone who samples anal play experiences this. The anus does not widen naturally like a vagina. If you persevere past the first couple of minutes, the discomfort will eventually turn to pleasure.

Anal sex offers depths of pleasure in both men/women. It is often deemed as a naughty "out of bounds" area, but it can heighten the sexual relationship of any couple. Ask a man about anal sex and I'm sure he will respond with curiosity. The fantasy of making love to a tight hole can push his mind into delirium.

If you are ready to create a memorable experience, allow anal sex to dominate your sexual agenda. For anal sex enthusiasts who feel ready to get kinky, read the following tips:

- **Use Condoms**: Always have a packet of condoms handy before you decide to experiment with anal sex. The anus is full of rich nerve endings, which makes this area prone to tears easily. If a penis or sex toy is inserted into a tight anus, chances are it will tear and bleed. If this occurs, the anal tissue is already damaged and could lead to sexually transmitted diseases (STDs), if your partner does not wear protection. If you hate condoms, attend a sexual health clinic together to be tested for STDs and HIV. Ensure you are both one hundred percent safe before experimenting in this area without protection. HIV results may take up to six months to provide a result of either positive or negative, so try to use protection until then.

- **Plan Ahead**: I love spontaneous foreplay, but anal sex is an exception. Anal sex should always be planned ahead, if possible. Buy condoms and shower or bathe beforehand. Clean all sex toys, empty the bladder, and avoid a heavy meal. Take a couple of psyllium husks with 250ml of water thirty minutes before a meal to flush out the colon. Alternatively, warm water with lemon juice is also a fantastic colon cleanser. Eat something light and nutritious, e.g. fruit or rice cakes. Taking psyllium husks or drinking warm water with lemon is an easier option than performing an enema.

- **Lubricant**: It is impossible to have comfortable anal sex without a large dose of lubricant. Unlike the vagina, the anus does not lubricate juices naturally. Feces should not be viewed as lubricants, nor should they been seen if the bowels are empty. Use an entire bottle of lubricant if it eases the discomfort of a penis or sex toy inserted into this tight hole.

- **Experiment**: If anal sex is a new area for you both, use fingers and sex toys, or ask your partner to rim the area with his/her tongue before penetration of the anus. This allows you to experience what it will feel like when the anus expands. The first minute may feel discomforting, but is rarely painful. If you persevere, this distress will transfer into pleasure.

- **Go Slowly**: You must respect your partner's comfort before experimenting with anal sex. Do not attempt to penetrate his/her ass like you would a vagina. This area is very sensitive and prone to tears. Listen for his/her moans of feedback. Are they moans of pleasure or pain? Have your partner's moans quietened because of distress? For women, if you dislike the experience, do not continue to please a partner. If you want respect, you must communicate your levels of comfort to your partner. Alternatively, penetrate the anus slowly until s/he states otherwise. If you remain patient during anal sex, your partner is more likely to relax and enjoy the sensation. Keep the area wet and slippery with lubrication.

- **Feedback**: It is important to give your partner feedback during the act, or discuss the issues where you feel concern beforehand. If you do not disclose this information, the early discomfort and resistance will play upon your mind. If you enjoy the sensations, encourage your partner to penetrate you harder/quicker/deeper. Moaning is a good form of feedback, but also spell out your enjoyment with explicit phases to spur on your partner. Discomforting moans often sound the same as pleasurable moans; so enquire with your partner about his/her pleasure during this intimate act.

- **Anal Toys**: Experiment with small vibrating dildos or anal beads throughout foreplay. During anal sex, it feels delightful to insert a vibrating bullet into the vagina to tickle the inside of the testicles. This also satisfies the female g-spot. Try this move if you wish to give your partner a memorable session.

- **Shower**: Wipe the area clean before anal sex, or if you plan to rim his/her ass with your tongue, always shower to ensure the area is pristinely clean, and also to avoid infection.

- **Strap-on Sex**: A lot of men are curious about the g-spot situated in the anus and will often ask a partner to penetrate them with a strap on. Ensure that you use a condom, a lot of lubricant, and go slowly, always enquiring to find out if he enjoys the pleasure and pace.

SEXUAL AIDS

BENEFITS OF SEX AND ORGASM

Sex and orgasms work to increase vitality, reduce stress, enhance pleasure, and maintain a healthy mind and body. Regular orgasms also work to strip off up to ten years. When natural endorphins—more potent than morphine—release during orgasm, they relieve pain, calm anxiety, and act as a preventative toward insomnia and depression.

A long masturbation or sex session burns many calories, reducing the craving for unhealthy foods and even nicotine. This is due to the elevated levels of the hormone, serotonin—the happy hormone, which releases during all sexual activity. Anti-depressants also work to raise the levels of serotonin in the brain, but now that you have the knowledge, would you choose to take conventional drugs for the same effect?

If your sole aim is to lose weight and tone up the muscles, try to have energetic sex regularly in a variety of positions to tone the problem areas. The longer the muscles are contracted, the stronger and more toned they will become.

During orgasm, a number of chemical reactions occur in the body. Before climax, DHEA—a natural steroid found in the body—increases beyond its regular levels. After its release, this natural hormone improves the heart and brain functions, boosts the immune system, metabolizes fat, and improves the texture and tone of the skin.

Women have a naturally high level of estrogen, and regular sex can help to protect the heart. In turn, sex also acts as a preventative against Alzheimer's disease and osteoporosis. Like any other exercise performed, sex and orgasms get the heart pumping and also boost the immune system. Unbelievably, sex is also a natural antihistamine and helps asthmatics and hay fever sufferers.

Real orgasms release endorphins to reduce stress, anxiety, and fear-based thoughts. Throughout daily life, our mind and body undergo physical and psychological challenges, most of which trigger anxiety and stress. Sex and masturbation work together to create a feeling of ecstasy through orgasm.

In women, an orgasm prevents menstrual cramps, breast pain, and also burns a hundred calories, on average. Man made painkillers of course help to block pain, but the body can become susceptible to drugs and a higher dose is often required to ease the same symptoms. Treat your body to a real orgasm and release your body's natural painkillers—endorphins. Your natural endorphins are stronger than morphine, and leave a pleasant calming effect on both the body and mind.

Anti-aging moisturizers are expensive, and I believe there are cheaper ways to prevent aging. I repeat the affirmation, "I am getting younger and younger every day." The mind doesn't know your current age, so if you continue to state a phrase, it will deliver its message to the brain and work its magic. However you must believe in what you are stating as there is no point saying a positive phrase, then letting your ego state, "What the hell are you saying you old crony."

There are thousands of anti-wrinkle creams, strong retinal products for the over fifties, and eye products available, but none of them can give you a glow like sex can. In order to get that illuminating glow that will turn others envious, manifest your time and energy into sex, masturbation, and orgasms. Sex is naturally anti-aging, but it is better to experiment with its pleasure regularly, for best effects.

Aging is caused through mind over matter. If you believe that you are going to age, your mind will give you exactly what you focus upon. Of course, we all age, but you can slow down the aging process by simply changing your mindset to think in the opposite way. Try it. It's free and the mind is the most powerful tool in the world, which can positively influence all areas of your life.

In my personal opinion, sex and orgasms—when used as regular exercise—is one of the best preventatives of stress, which is a huge degenerative ager. Stress is debilitating to the body and ages it both internally and externally. The depressing news and manipulative media spread so much fear, and it eventually catches hold of us all. Try not to live in the past or the future; the present holds so much power. Turn back the hands of time with regular masturbation, sex, and orgasms.

TELEPATHIC SUGGESTION

Did you know that it is possible to influence anyone you meet through the power of your mind? Be honest with yourself. Have you ever fed a thought to someone and s/he played upon your suggestion? If this worked, even if the move was only small (like an itch of the nose or slight movement), you were successful in telepathically suggesting something beyond his/her awareness.

Everyone has psychic abilities, but they require time and effort to develop to the heights where you do not have to think about it to use the gift. Nevertheless, we often tune into different states of consciousness during reality. Daydreaming and meditation are just two heightened state of consciousness.

To telepathically suggest something sexually, you must focus on the thought, visualize it, and continue to state it hundreds of times to ensure its success. This is great for first dates when you want him/her to kiss you. Attraction is psychic in itself.

How many of you ignore communication before you get kinky with another? For instance, have you ever had a nasty fight with your partner, but felt aroused throughout the experience? Fights are not pleasant, but the make up sex is worth the wait.

During the relationship with my first boyfriend, we had a lot of verbal fights. He was a possessive man and didn't want me to have a social life with my friends. As a Muslim, he was teetotal, until that all changed one night when he was too stressed to do much else. I loved the sound of his voice, even when he hated me. I wanted to make love to him so much, which is the test of true love I guess. I used to feed sexual thoughts through telepathy into his mind, and I always got my own way. The sex was often better than normal.

During an argument with your partner, take a moment to reflect. Do your genitals speak the truth about your attraction to him/her? Do you communicate regularly with your partner? Communication is important. Instead of watching a movie, turn off the TV, light a candle, focus full attention on your partner, and get to know him/her further. Sit apart from each other so you can maintain eye contact. You do not need to discuss sex, talk about anything. Try to make a connection with his/her mind. Make flirty telepathic suggestion, e.g. "Pounce on me," or "Give me the fuck of my life tonight." These are just some of the rude thoughts shooting through my head during first dates or relationships.

Of course, telepathic suggestion is possible if your partner is open minded, and most of what you communicate daily is often subconscious through telepathy. For example, if you are thinking of a song and it plays on the radio, or you think about someone and they suddenly call or appear. This is no coincidence; this is the power of the mind at work.

Instead of stripping your partner and using your tongue and fingers to arouse his/her nerve endings, focus on feeding his/her mind with sexual thoughts. If you practice for long enough, you will turn him/her into a human sex toy who will obey your every command.

Telepathic suggestion[54] is just one type of Extra Sensory Perception, and everyone has this magic power within. It requires work, focus, and patience. Do not try to force ESP as it often comes naturally. It is possible to influence another person by planting sexual thoughts in his/her mind.

Telepathy is within our reality daily. If you watch the news, the negativity can sink into your mind altering your mood. The economy is a huge example. The world is abundant, and there is more than enough money in the world for everyone to live comfortably. What you think about you create, so if you allow the media to manipulate you with negativity and then start to worry or focus on fear, you no longer have the power over your own free will. The media telepathically suggest that you think negatively. No positive experience will appear in the mind of a low vibrating or negative person.

However, you have the free reign over your mind, and you can change it with positive thoughts and action. You have phenomenal power within your mind and can develop your psychic abilities to the point where you can influence another person. Build up this power through meditation and ask your Higher Self[55] to enter your energy field. The answer will often manifest quickly, especially if the mind is open to suggestion, or you may receive an answer through your dreams. If you are especially open minded you might receive an affirmative answer through number synchronicity. Alternatively, an answer could appear on the radio, TV, or while reading a newspaper/book.

The Higher Self is always trying to grab your attention, and the gut instincts you receive are from your Higher Self. How many of you have often said, "Oh I knew I should have followed my instinct." This is because you failed to trust your Higher Self. It is always trying to link you to the most positive choices that will influence *your* life.

When you are walking alone, you may get the urge to walk one-way and not the other. This is your Higher Self also working to protect you from harm. However, there are certain instances when your intuition is not in sync with your mind. This is often due to alcohol or mind-altering drugs.

In one of my previous jobs where I worked in administration, I got the hunch to leave. When two bosses spoke to me like a piece of shit on their high heel, and I got a bad "vibe" about the building, I couldn't ignore my instinct a second longer. Of course, I worried about money and all the other crap that plants fear in the mind, but eventually I took a leap of faith and never looked back.

If you feel too nervous to try telepathic suggestion on your partner for fear that it could harm him/her, why don't you try it on someone else? It could be something daft like, "itch your nose," or "look behind you." Once you notice that your influence has worked on a stranger or work colleague, try a positive sexual suggestion on your partner. If this works, keep it a secret from your partner as telepathy does interfere with free will. However, continue working on this telepathy and it will gradually strengthen, like everything other skill.

Although there is no scientific knowledge of Extra Sensory Perception, do you need proof for the "unknown" to contain truth? There is a Higher Power around us daily. It wants to work with us and through us to enhance our life and that of others.

PORN

The porn industry is one of the richest in the world and continues to grow through adult magazines, movies, fetish clothing, sex toys, pheromones, and sexual enhancers like the infamous Viagra. Sex is visually exciting, but it often comes at a price! To watch a sexy female stripping off her clothes or participating in a long visually exciting blowjob session, one must first pay to view the experience.

Nymphomaniacs who crave a penis pumping her tight ass during anal sex, or two best friends experimenting in a lesbian romp are just two of the hundreds of thousands of scenes on offer in pornographic movies.

Women enjoy reading explicit magazines or watching a visually exciting movie with her partner. Many couples are able to feel horny while watching a porn movie together. Jealous partners may pull a face at the thought of his/her partner viewing porn, but it does not need to be taken seriously. Instead, view it in a positive light.

Men are naturally visual. The hint of flesh or view of explicit words is enough to cause an erection in men. All men must remember the importance of sharing their sexual needs with a partner, including whether or not you crave porn to grow sexually aroused. Do not feel embarrassed. Your partner must first learn to understand your needs and want to put your pleasure first. The view of naked curves in movies and magazines drives out the hungry desire in men. Women can easily take part in the action by dressing in provocative clothing, participating in fantasies, and writing erotica.

Some women may feel hurt or even threatened to find out that their partner views porn or naked magazines in private. Instead, try to be understanding and recognize his needs. Men/women are very different and far too many misunderstandings can occur through mistrust, jealousy, and lack of communication.

It takes courage for a man to admit of a love for porn, but it could then turn into a guilty secret if it is not disclosed to a partner. Be honest with your partner. Porn is not viewed as cheating if you are honest about your sexual fetish, but if your partner then finds a collection of movies hidden under the bed, the situation is very likely to cause her concern. In this scene, it is essential to communicate with your partner to discuss your sexual needs.

Why do you or your partner view porn? Is it for the sight of naked women/men, the dirty rampant sex, teasing blowjobs, or perhaps all three? If you know that your partner views porn on a regular basis, but s/he remains secretive of that fact, how does it make you feel inward? Sick, envious, or relieved.

The majority of women view porn as a form of cheating. However, it is important to note WHY he views porn or reads dirty magazines. Is it a form of tension release because you refuse him sex, or does he need to view explicit images or words to reach arousal? The former could be a positive step when viewed from outside the triangle. During long-term relationships and marriage, it is important to retain intimacy. Couples who remain together are able to maintain their sexual attraction by spending time together, and/or experimenting with new techniques.

Of course, a relationship built on honesty will build a strong and satisfying sex life. Sex is private, and no one else need know about what you and your partner get up to in the bedroom. It is natural to want to experiment sexually, especially if you are in a long-term relationship or married. Pornography is a form of visual foreplay, and most men/women find it pleasurable and satisfying.

The porn industry continues to grow, but not everyone would like to view a stick thin longhaired model with neat vaginal lips and a tight ready-to-penetrate ass. In reality, men love every inch of the female anatomy. Most women view the sight of their vaginal lips as unattractive, but a high proportion of men love the sight and scent. Cosmetic surgery now allows the vaginal lips to be snipped to neaten the area, and porn stars often have cosmetically enhanced genitals. The need for perfection can cause obsession in women who are paranoid about the size of their lips, then disallow their partner to perform oral sex because of this growing fear. However, you must remember that the world would be a very boring place if everyone looked the same. It's time to embrace every part of your body, including your genitals.

Rather than put yourself through the pain of genital cosmetic surgery, book a salon appointment for a Hollywood wax to feel better about your body. Your partner loves every inch of you. I agree that the female vagina looks wrinkly and weird, but to a huge number of men it is a heavenly sight.

Cosmetic surgery can tighten and neaten the vagina, but the same is achievable without a distinguishable alteration as drastic as surgery. Kegal exercises train the pelvic floor muscles, and every time you stop yourself from urinating you are in control of this muscle. If you have never before worked this muscle, it may feel uncomfortable at first. I personally hate kegal exercises and prefer to masturbate.

During orgasm, the vagina spasms between five to ten seconds. While you can feel the contractions of the vagina during kegal exercises, the waves of orgasm distract your mind from these same uncomfortable sensations.

The female figure is another example of how the porn industry view perfection. I estimate that many female porn models have to retain their petite figures as part of the contract. This is unfortunate for the normal women of the world, like myself, who store a little meat on the bones.

Perfectionist men prefer a "trophy bird" on their arm. They are often extremely shallow and never look beyond image. Insecurities can also push some men to focus on perfection. Often the right partner will come along, perhaps very different from his usual choice of woman, but the illusion of looks misleads him into another disastrous relationship with a high maintenance woman to match his mirror image. True happiness lies in the self. If you are content with yourself, looks and image should not take high priority. Your partner should be a mirror image of your thoughts and attractive qualities.

A curvy figure between the sizes of ten to sixteen is the average figure that men desire. Sexiness derives from confidence. If you are happy with your figure and show it off in daring clothes, men will view an incredibly sexy woman.

The next time you are out with your female friends, look around the room at sexy women, and study their moves. The same rule applies to men. If you carry an air of mystery and confidence, your energy field becomes magnetically attractive to the opposite sex, or the same sex if you are homosexual.

Women often feel disappointed or betrayed to know that a partner watches porn to view a nine-inch penis pounding a petite model with huge breasts and zero body fat. Those kinky fantasies can rise to another level by continuing to watch porn in secret. Perhaps he wants to view a sexually exciting woman, as he craves this in reality. The thought of sleeping with a woman with no sexual inhibitions is the ultimate turn on for men.

Men are visual and need to express those desires by watching porn or reading horny stories/magazines. Do not feel disappointed by his behavior. Porn is a natural necessity, which allows him to become quite deviant.

Have you ever considered getting kinky with your partner for a short home video? There is a huge selection of quality mobile phones available with built in video recorders which record excellent footage. Alternatively, use the movie feature on a digital camera to record your dirty exploits.

Many couples still feel guilty about stepping out of the ordinary bedroom to explore experimentation elsewhere. Recording a sex scene may feel daunting at first, but remember that only you and your partner are starring in the scene. Let go of fear and embarrassment, and embrace your sexuality.

Turn an erotic scene into a positive sexual experience that remains memorable. Imagine how it would feel to walk into work feeling ultra happy, while your colleagues wonder what has caused your beaming smile? Recording a short pornographic movie on your phone is only for the brave, but will remain with you always. Add a sim code lock onto your phone if it is ever lost or stolen. In this way, no one can view your private videos, even after the phone has been unlocked.

Lose your inhibitions for one night only. Do not be shy about stripping off your clothes. Give your partner the phone or digital camera, and let him/her record your slow teasing strip. Make a hot movie you will both enjoy watching regularly.

If a porn movie arouses your partner, a homemade sex movie will offer the same with the added bonus that it remains very personal and authentic. Watch it regularly and design some new moves, which you know will look great on a homemade sex movie.

If you dislike the thought of your partner watching porn or reading explicit magazines, you need to take charge by becoming a porn star for the night. Experimenting with homemade movies also displays the fact that you have no sexual inhibitions. This will turn you into a Goddess, unleashing a side of you that is not often visible in the bedroom.

EROTICA

Erotica is a fun way to arouse the genitals through the power of explicit words. Many women prefer to read romantic erotica with a clean storyline and a happy-ever-after ending, but other women prefer to read explicit content. The author's mind creates the storyline, and s/he then adds romance and sex to titillate the reader. Erotica is available online or through the larger high street bookshops. Stage 1 requires a book of steamy erotica. When you both feel comfortable and in the mood to get kinky, try this fun foreplay.

Stage 1: Set a romantic theme with music, essential oils, candles, and dimmed lighting. Remain fully clothed and ensure there are no distractions. Turn off your cell phone, lock the door, and focus one hundred percent energy on your partner. Try to step into character as you read the first chapter aloud to your partner. Short explicit tales are the perfect tool to use to arouse your partner. Alternatively, set aside time to read an explicit novella together.

When it is time for your partner to read the next chapter aloud, close your eyes and focus on the character. Try to feel every emotion s/he experiences throughout the story. If sexual urges flood the mind, allow them to take hold. Feel good about yourself. If the female character is a sexy mistress, imagine how it would feel to step into her shoes. Does she moan or talk dirty throughout the scene? Mimic those moves to alter your partner's mindset and genitals.

Reading erotica together can be mind-blowing foreplay for couples who employ its elements. It is fun, horny, and different. You may reach a point in your explicit tale where you and your partner are fully aroused. If so, move onto stage 2. Reading to your partner is very different than reading alone. Be patient while you are reading or listening to the tale. There may be a stage where you want to rip off your partner's clothes, but remain patient and try to close off the power of your sexual mind. Continue to build a level of sexual tension.

Stage 2: It's time to work with your creative mind to write a short explicit tale together. Visualize the fantasy you would like to become a reality, the same that your inhibitions would not allow you to carry further in the past, and put all your emotions and senses into the scene.

Are you normally a reserved person? If so, step into the role of a minx who can easily seduce her partner. Keep the story explicit and allow the surge of sexual energy pumping through your mind to arouse your genitals.

Do you choose to become a professional dominatrix who leaves a memorable impression on every man she meets? If so, step into character and dress the part. Fantasy or fetish clothing can be purchased online from most sex shops.

Perhaps your partner is a naughty doctor who takes advantage of his patients? In reality, this is a dangerous game to play, but as part of your erotic tale it remains taboo and sexy. Write about scenes of fantasy you have yet to experience with your partner.

Banish your shy side and guilt with deep breaths to bring you back into the now moment. Use sexy thoughts to affect your sexuality. Create a steamy scene and let your body experience the pleasure it deserves.

Allow your thoughts to dominate your creativity. If a sexual thought is beyond your comprehension, speak it, write it, and/or discuss the scene thoroughly with your partner. Once the scene is set, and the foreplay is described in intimate detail, move onto stage 3.

Stage 3: By this point after reading and writing erotica together, you should be feeling quite horny and ready to play out the scene in reality. Do not waste time by waiting for your partner to initiate sex, simply pounce! Does the scene feel the same as any other routine sex session, or do you now experience fireworks?

Act out the story in reality. If the scene takes place in the cinema, visit the movies together, and become a filthy dynamic duo who are almost caught in the act. Try to remain in character to continue with the fun elements.

Erotica is playful and opens up the sexual mind to experimentation. I would say that the only downside to erotica is the required time you must set aside. Experiment with erotica only when your mind is free of stress and you have the time available. You must also be in the right frame of mind to step into this realm of hot fantasy. Use your creative mind to develop a sexy scene in which to star. Writing erotica could soon feel natural, if you practice often enough.

SEX TOYS

Sex toys vary in both size and degrees of intensity. Huge dildos are available in black, white, and deep brown to imitate a human penis. For men, lifelike vaginas suck in the penis—perfect for adventurous males.

If the toy of choice is an anal stimulator, first experiment with anal beads to gently rim the area before full insertion. Women who experience no pleasure with large dildos may find the smaller vibrating eggs to be perfect for the clit. The rabbit is also a pleasant choice because of its attached ears, which stimulate the clitoris; and the large rubber dildo satisfies the g-spot. Toys are perfect to use alone or with a partner to heighten the senses.

A sex toy is the perfect weapon to use during masturbation. If you have the confidence and attitude, toys will enhance any sexual act. Couples with an intention to add sex toys to the relationship will experience heightened pleasure. An example would be if your partner has asked you to tickle his testicles with a vibrating egg. Give him what he wants. Take a deep breath, choose selective explicit words to excite him into the spontaneous scene, and create his sexual hunger using your fingers, tongue, and kinky sex toys. Go one step further by including oral sex, which will keep him on red alert and make it feel like a real dominatrix session.

Most individuals feel limited in his/her oral sex abilities, or the thought of performing this act creates nervous tension and paranoia. Sex toys now exist primarily to provide that direct stimulation for the genitals. A cheeky vibrator humming against the clitoris, a vibrating egg tickling your partner's testicles, or a soft jelly toy stimulated over the nipples can push nervous excitement into blissful ecstasy.

The tongue is the strongest muscle in the human body and has multiple uses. Without a tongue, we would be unable to talk, lick, taste, and stimulate the skin. The tongue produces saliva to keep the teeth and gums healthy. It is the perfect sex toy. Stimulate your partner's skin with a lick of your tongue. Plant erotic kisses on his/her mouth, lick over and around the nipples, and wet your partner's genitals. The tongue excites the penis, clitoris, nipples, Adam's apple, and many other hot erogenous zones. Whichever area you choose to focus your energies, the experienced pleasure will remain a prevalent memory in your partner's mind. S/he may wriggle and moan, or the constant stimulations could drive out an unseen sexual force.

However, there is a downside when using the tongue—dehydration. If you plan to seduce your partner with your tongue, drink a couple of glasses of water beforehand. If your throat becomes dry throughout foreplay, dehydration will continue to steal moisture from the tongue. In this instance, use a sex toy to furnish pleasure on your partner.

Sex toys are not the only insertions for the male and female genitals. There are other fun tools to use during sex and foreplay, e.g. heated massage oils, melting chocolates (for the body), sexy lingerie, or flavored condoms. Sex shops sell thousands of vibrators; fetish clothing, lingerie, rude shaped chocolates, sex games, and edible massage oils.

Does your partner fantasize an image of you dressed in latex? If yes, visit a sex shop or purchase a sexy outfit online. Sex shops sell a variety of naughty uniforms, including doctors and nurses, dominatrix, and rubber clothing for fetishists.

Communicate with your partner to find out what s/he would like to gain from the addition of sex toys. If you are clear in your sexual vision you will find what you need in a sex shop. If you feel embarrassed about visiting a high street sex shop, visit one of the many online sex shops instead. They often have affiliate schemes so you can make a little extra cash if you promote their products on your website. Other sex shops offer a discount on first orders.

Relaxation is required to enhance sexual pleasure. Try solo sex, mutual masturbation, or oral sex with your partner. Deep breaths and meditation can heighten any sexual experience, deepen levels of confidence, and enhance your awareness of thought.

It is impossible to climax if the mind is filled with worry, anxiety, and tension. Kundalini[56] energy remains asleep in the lower spine, but immediately awakens during sexual activity and orgasm. Meditation and chanting can awaken the powerful Kundalini energy in a subtle way. Orgasms can never be forced; they happen only when the sexual mind is ready to set off that electrical spark of pleasure.

The Ultimate Sex Toy: Sex toys exist primarily to give and receive sexual pleasure, but the most powerful sex toy in existence is the human mind. To heighten any sexual experience, use your mind to focus on the part of the body receiving attention.

Would you agree that it is near impossible to focus one hundred percent attention and have multi-orgasms with more than one person at the same time? A sexual connection can develop only if you already share a strong bond with your partner.

Most individuals settle for a partner who is incompatible with them in many ways, including sexually. Why should life focus on settling for second best? You deserve to experience fun, love, and fireworks, but it is your choice to seek this sexual pleasure with a mutually compatible partner.

Use natural pheromones to enhance your sexual scent, which offers you the highest chance of attracting a well-matched partner. If you were lucky enough to find that special spark with a partner, why would you need to look elsewhere?

You must work together with a partner to develop a satisfying sex life. Is there a particular foreplay technique that you both like/dislike? There is always a fun way to turn disappointment into satisfaction through communication and experimentation.

Learn to love offering selfless pleasure to your partner. An erotic kiss arouses you both. Stroking enhances the pleasure of both the giver and the receiver, especially after first contact with soft skin.

Sex toys are fun to use on special occasions, but the hottest erogenous zones are the skin and the mind. Used together, these hot spots heighten the pleasure of any sexual activity, as well as enhancing orgasm. Work with your partner to connect soulfully. Talk, kiss, caress, massage, and/or stimulate his/her skin, and fully concentrate on the sensations you feel from your partner during foreplay through the power of your sexual mind.

Toys are fun and pleasurable to use in selective scenes, but the mind contains all of the magic tricks you will ever need for sexual satisfaction. Turn on your genitals in a second through the power of your mind. When your partner attacks your genitals with his/her fingers and tongue, release any tension in the body through deep breaths, and remain focused on the projected pleasure. Display feedback through shallow breaths, fervent moans, and a writhing body.

What could be more inspirational than finding a sexual connection with a partner, without the use of toys or stimulants; every moment heightened through your mind?

FUN SEX TIPS

TIPS FOR WOMEN

Masturbate: How can you expect to reach orgasm if you have no idea of how you like to be touched? Experiment with your fingers, lubricants, and sex toys while visualizing a hot fantasy. In this way, you will find it easier to free the potency contained within your sexual mind. When your mind feels excitement the genitals feel it too.

Only through masturbation will you learn the depth of contact required on your clitoris to reach orgasm. This is important, especially throughout oral sex. As I have stated numerous times throughout this guide, masturbation is NOT a sin.

Men embrace a sexual partner who experiences oral sex with or without his help? You can develop this a step further by allowing him to watch you in action. With the latter, a level of confidence is required, but it helps in three ways. (1) It shows your partner how you like to be touched, (2) builds your inner confidence and develops sexual prowess, and (3), turns you into a Goddess to be worshipped.

Show him exactly how gentle or firmly you crave his touch. Moan, wriggle, and throw back your head in ecstasy during masturbation. Do all the things necessary to illustrate how you want his tongue to lick you during oral sex.

Research conducted on masturbation found that up to seventy percent of women fake an orgasm once during their life. Fifteen percent of women fake it eighty percent of the time. Nine and a half percent of women like to fake an orgasm occasionally, which leaves the final half a percent who never fake an orgasm. These statistics prove that there are a lot of unsatisfied women worldwide. Men reading this may find it hard to accept, but time, devotion, and solid effort is the key to satisfying your partner.

If your partner is selfish when it comes to oral sex, the only positive thing you can teach him is how you like to touch yourself. Practice masturbation in front of a mirror, or video yourself in action. If this is the only thing you can teach a man sexually, it is vital to spread this knowledge. The sign of a real orgasm is clear to see—her clitoral hood retracts, her vagina spontaneously contracts, her body shakes, and her pupils dilate. Look for these signs in a woman during her climax.

A real orgasm is one of the best experiences in the world, so why would you want to fake it to satisfy a partner? You are doing nothing to boost his ego. If he knew the truth, I'm sure it would mortify him. Unconditional love and orgasms are infinite. Not only do women love the experience of blissful orgasmic pleasure melting away stress and muscle tension, but he feels every emotion too!

The sexual pleasure in both partners multiplies to incredible heights when he knows how you satisfy you through oral sex or masturbation. Teach him about the pleasures you crave through solo sex, and allow him to watch you so that he discovers the level of intensity required for you to reach orgasm. If you find this difficult, practice first in front of a mirror, or down a couple of shots of vodka for courage. Deep breaths also help to relax the mind and body.

The hottest sex toy of all is the human mind. Take your time during masturbation, but never rush or try to force an orgasm, as this could create tension or even make it impossible to orgasm. Visualize a sexy image—one of which could be the sight of your partner rubbing his dick softly, while he watches you stroking your genitals.

Once you approach the realization of how effortless it is to achieve orgasm, the hunger to reach those same heights will dominate your mind. If he is successfully able to satisfy you through masturbation, oral sex, intercourse, and even passionate kisses, you have no need to look elsewhere.

Orgasm: It is possible to strengthen the pelvic floor muscles naturally. One such device to achieve this is via a kegal toning device. This inserts into the vagina and the surrounding muscles clench and release the device. If the thought of using that simple device puts you off, you will be pleased to know that there is an easier way to develop a tighter pussy—through orgasm.

During climax, endorphins flood the body bestowing warmth and satisfaction, whilst the vagina sporadically contracts on average five to ten times. None of the pelvic floor tightening exercises are felt because of the natural vaginal response throughout orgasm.

Experiment with both fingers and toys to reach orgasm. Climax is easily achievable through foreplay, sexual intercourse, and masturbation. A multi-orgasmic side may also unleash through basic foreplay moves, e.g. touch and kissing, in other women.

Pheromones: These invisible sexual scents play cupid to attract a compatible partner in order to mate healthy children. Perfumes and aftershaves smell lush, but they are synthetic, expensive, and mask the natural pheromones found in the human body. If you allowed your pheromones to work their magic, I am sure it would be surprising to note the sexual chemistry between you and your next partner.

Essential oils and alcohol are the main ingredients of perfume and aftershave. You can, however, make your own perfume by diluting essential oils in carrier oil, e.g. jojoba, and allow them to affect your central nervous system. When mixed with alcohol, essential oils lose their natural potency.

Synthetic pheromones sprays can be purchased online in sex shops, although I would estimate they are not cheap. The truth that the powerful pharmaceutical industries do not want each of us to know is that natural attracting pheromones are found within everyone. Animals cope well attracting prey, yet why does most of the world believe s/he requires additional tools of attraction to attract sexual prey? If left alone, the invisible chemical messengers get to work on finding you a well-matched partner to match your DNA. However, when the body is masked with synthetic fragrances, the body undergoes difficulty in seeking a true sexual chemistry with another.

Natural pheromones are found in sexual lubricants, semen, urine, and perspiration. Experiment with your natural scent by rubbing the ointment of your choice on pulse points, e.g. the wrists, inside of elbow, nape of the neck, and around the belly button, etc. If you remain patient, I guarantee that you will meet a partner whom you share a strong sexual bond with and who also takes you to incredible sexual heights.

The media or fragrance industry will not speak this truth, or society states that it is better to smell good, as it denotes success, popularity, attractiveness, and self-worth. Open up your eyes to the illusion that is surrounding you in the current world and experiment with this new knowledge, which has always been in existence, yet not promoted to the masses.

For the majority of you reading this chapter, the thought of dabbing the pulse points with urine or sexual lubricant may sound unnatural and disgusting. I might be the first to set a worldwide trend! You have free will and your own mind; you can make your own choice. Celebrities are paid a huge amount of money to promote products so that consumers buy the item. This includes food, skincare, perfume, financial sectors, insurance, and music.

You have the power within to attract a soul mate. If synthetic fragrances did not exist, your pheromones would have no choice but to work 24/7 on your behalf to attract partners who can offer you long lasting sexual satisfaction. Since I found out about this fact, I have used my own pheromones on pulse points to attract hot lovers. Trust me, it works like magic!

If you would prefer to enhance your natural invisible scent, make your own fragrance with a little olive oil and a couple of drops of the natural aphrodisiacs, vanilla and ylang ylang essential oils. This scent will penetrate the deepest layer of the skin—the dermis, therefore affecting the nervous system, while making you smell luscious to your partner. Essential oils are very potent, and just one drop of natural perfume will last far longer than masking synthetic fragrances. Vanilla is a well-known aphrodisiac and is especially arousing to men.

Give Feedback And Move: Wriggle or moan your partner's name to display any form of feedback through foreplay and lovemaking. If you remain quiet or shy, it may be difficult for your partner to "read" your pleasure. Dirty phrases may be all s/he craves from you, but an eager moan or whispered sentence describing your fulfilling ecstasy can build an intense connection between you both.

Do not lie underneath your partner like a lazy sack of spuds; MOVE! Most men crave the excitement of an adventurous woman. Display enthusiasm through moans, stimulating foreplay, or explicit words, and your partner will crave your newfound sexual energy. Men love any form of encouragement during sex, plus they also experience insecurities in the bedroom, like everyone else.

If you would love him to view you as a Goddess, all you need to do is to act and believe you are the only woman who can build and release his sexual gratification. This is not an ego-boost; it is appreciating your self-worth. Create his arousal with fun foreplay, and show off a new dominating side that illustrates no mercy when he tries to disobey you.

Release your natural pheromones during an energizing sexual workout and improve your fitness. Think of exciting places to make love, e.g. a rocking chair, unusual item of furniture, or during a raging storm etc. Sex does not always have to be performed in the bedroom. Once you open your mind to its potential, there will be no return to borderline sex.

Oral Sex: This selfless act creates intimacy between couples, although it is not for everyone. Oral sex is often given with the hope that it is returned, but many women do not enjoy fellatio.

Men like to watch a partner display enthusiasm during oral sex. Consider your partner's pleasure during oral sex and work toward that, rather than pull a discouraging face.

Oral sex burns many calories and is a fantastic workout for the face, especially when performed regularly. Fellatio also tones the chin, an area that can grow saggy as women grow older. With the huge variety of breast or chin toning creams, I have never understood how a cream can tone certain areas of the body without exercise. Oral sex is a great workout for the chin and will snip off any excess fat. A couple of sessions per week is sufficient exercise for the face and jaw line. Make eye contact with him throughout the intimate act, and he will be in awe of you.

Finally, if you can stomach semen, aim to swallow! Sperm is a great source of protein, vitamin C, and zinc, plus it contains very few calories. With a mouthful of semen, this act also gives you the advantage in experimental games, e.g. share a kiss full of cum. Although this may sound disgusting to some men, it is daring and different, especially to open-minded men.

TIPS FOR MEN

Technique: There are two types of men in the bedroom; those who like to pleasure a woman, and men who have no concern for a partner's pleasure after an orgasm. Some men are eager to satisfy a woman during intercourse. There are many books available today on how to become a bastard to women, adopting bad boy traits to attract a woman. No doubt these tips work, but you do not have to adopt an unnatural tendency to offer excitement to a partner.

There are similar books available for women on how to play hard to get to keep a man. Both varieties of books offer interesting facts, but at the end of the day all these techniques focus on game play. Men may not display as many romantic elements as women do in a relationship, but this does not signify that he is boring or unloving. Women naturally offer love toward a partner, and playing hard to get could be difficult for both parties. Men/women are equally fascinating.

Some men believe that hard sex equals gratification for both parties. If your partner feels content and displays a smile, all aspects of the relationship remain fine. A quickie feels sufficient on occasions, but women do not enjoy it all the time. Men must learn and understand women, just as women need to learn and understand men.

Women require multiple foreplay moves and sufficient time to convert sexual thoughts into arousal. Foreplay also helps a woman to feel sexually desired. A hard penis offers her satisfaction, but you must also build her levels of desire. Men love hard penetration, and most women too, but if you have no desire to pleasure her with anything other than a hard fuck, your sex life could falter. A quickie eases stress, releases endorphins, but may not fulfill her true sexual needs.

Men can become aroused quite easily through passionate kisses or any other foreplay move. The penis is an easy tool to stimulate. A sexy female who flaunts her figure on the street, or the view of a hot cleavage advertising a push up bra on a massive billboard could have an urgent effect on his penis.

A conversation about sex or a short read of erotica often causes a rush of blood to the penis. There are dozens of stimulants to create arousal in men. Sedentary men who smoke, take drugs, or those who are unsatisfied with their relationship could find it difficult to maintain an erection.

How do you know if you are sexually exciting in the bedroom? If you can easily stimulate your partner to create her orgasm, you are already viewed as a sex God through her eyes. If you have doubts about your performance, work with your partner to find out the level of desire and touch she craves. How does she like to be rubbed, kissed, and caressed during sex? Step out of the ordinary and help her to reach her peak of ecstasy.

Your partner may soon start to resent sex if she does not receive sufficient pleasure in the bedroom. However, she too has a role to play in communicating her arousal. Ask her directly or experiment with varied pressures until she is moaning with ecstasy. Some men can manage to work a woman into frenzy during sexual foreplay, but when intercourse transpires and she does not experience an orgasm, she fakes an orgasm to please her man. This does not create intimacy or a special sexual bond with a partner.

If you have no idea on how to push your sex life from ordinary to steaming hot, it could cause your partner to become quiet, unsatisfied, and seek pleasure elsewhere for simple tension release. Alternatively, she may just turn to masturbation. I am in no way relating that she would have an affair, but other tools may enter her life, including sex toys, online flirting games, or porno films. Women also enter horny periods throughout their life and seek alternative pleasures if they reach no fulfillment with a partner. To avoid this, try to remain enthusiastic about foreplay, and spend hours exciting her to the brink of orgasm.

Women can become great actresses in the moment, but instinctively she may know that a problem exists. In short-term relationships, sexual problems can subside, causing the original issue to fade. However, in long-term relationships, if the concern is not resolved, it could weaken your once strong relationship. This is not your fault. Ensure that your levels of communication remain robust.

Only through masturbation can a woman find out exactly what thoughts and images awaken her genitals. With self-confidence comes the confession of how she likes to stroke herself. A clitoral orgasm is very different from a vaginal or g-spot orgasm, so give her no excuse to fake another one ever again!

Why do women not discuss their sexual problems to a partner? The problem could derive from hormones, stress, or the fear of approaching the matter with a partner. If you wish to become her dream lover, communicate with her to find out her likes/dislikes, even if it takes a lot of time, patience, and effort on your part. This will prove your strength, commitment, and love for her.

Compliments: During courtship, a relationship is exciting and you cannot keep your hands off your partner in and out of the bedroom. She loves filling your mind with compliments, and you equally make her feel confident and sexually desired. Whether you have been together for four weeks, four months, four years, or forty years, look for ways to compliment her daily.

Do not take advantage of her and expect that a relationship requires no patience and effort from you; only the longest relationships survive with love, commitment, trust, and cherished time spent together. If you love your partner's legs, stroke them during a massage. If you love your partner's lips, give her a hot French kiss that will stimulate all of her nerve endings and awaken her genitals. Be spontaneous.

Show Affection And Cause Desire: Women are big lovers of touch and affection. Imagine that she is one hundred percent relaxed and lay naked on the bed. Run your fingertips delicately over her entire body to cause goose bumps. Experiment with this tip by using your fingers to gently stimulate the inside of your arm to feel how easily it can heighten the sense of touch.

Another perfect way to excite her in an instant is to run your nails slowly over her skin. Spend time on creating her desire, which will build a sexual yearn for her to crave more. With the knowledge of how important touch is to a woman, running both your hands down her entire body should feel an exhilarating practice. If you spot an instant change in her body—shallow breaths, flowing juices, a writhing body, and the sex "flush"—you are already building desire in her body and mind.

Continue this foreplay for five minutes without stimulating any of the hot erogenous zones she is desperate for you to touch. Her arousal will build and build, driving her totally wild. She may scream your name or writhe like a woman possessed by an entity. Work your fingertips up to her breast, but refrain from stimulating the nipples.

Massage her breasts with the palm of your hand and fingertips. For extra stimulation, lick and kiss around her breasts, but do not touch the nipple—even though they look delicious and suckable. Caress beneath, to the side, and above them, but not directly upon them.

These purposeful moves will drive her crazy for you. By creating desire in her for you to stimulate her nipples, you retain control. A little thought and attention directed to specific areas of her body will cause her instant desire, while building excitement in you. Listen to her body, watch her moves, and she will let you know exactly when to take charge of her sexuality.

Move onto her clitoris, and arouse it with your hard penis. She should already be on red alert for your moves and be offering feedback in various forms. Tell her that your penis is willing and ready to enter her at any time. Build her desire until she begs for penetration. The direct aim is to cause her desperation, but self-control is required on your part.

When she requests sex early on, refrain—if possible to drive her extra crazy. Incredible sex is worth the wait. Even when she screams at you to fuck her, continue to rub your penis directly over her clitoris. Her arousal and orgasmic pleasure is building to an insane height, and it is *you* who has caused her in depth frustration.

Go one step further by slipping inside her a couple of inches before using your self-control to pull out. Continue with this foreplay to build up her levels of desire for you. Push it into her wet slit a couple more inches and then pull out again. Try to discourage pushing your entire length inside her. Every time you pull out, rub your penis lightly over her clit. Make sure not to continue rubbing this area as lush as it feels; it could cause her premature orgasm.

Continue to tease her no matter how frustrated you feel. The longer you can maintain this "creating desire" foreplay, the further intense both your orgasms will feel. When she finally surrenders to you, penetrate her and speed up your lovemaking. This will push her over the edge with a powerful orgasm. Listen to her body during foreplay. Look for enthusiastic moans and the shivers up and down your spine as she screams your name. The excitement of building her into such a frustrated state will ensure you explode with an equally potent orgasm.

If you love to tease her and wish to take it a step further, taunt her with foreplay. Make love to her until you both reach the peak of ecstasy, then stop and cuddle. Make love hours later, or wait until the morning. The next time your bodies rub together, she will be craving you so much that foreplay will be the last thing on her mind.

Note: Resist giving her what she wants. Do not grope her breasts or tweak her nipples during foreplay, although it may be difficult to restrain yourself. In the early stages, do not caress her clitoris; this could turn off her pleasure switch far too quickly.

Kinky women DO love hard sex and crave their nipples pinched and sucked hard, so they are an exception. If you know your partner inside and out, try this teasing foreplay to build up her levels of desire for you.

Remain in control throughout and let the foreplay drive you both nuts. Use your mind to focus on the thoughts and feelings she plants in your body and mind as you arouse her body, and she will give in with a horny release.

Role-Play: Live out a real fantasy. Try to surprise your partner by asking her to meet you at her favorite bar or restaurant. When she arrives, pretend that you are meeting for the first time. Keep her on edge with flirty glances. When she realizes the scope of the game, her tension will subside and hot sex will be the end-result. If the role-play fantasy causes a fight, remember that make-up sex is worth the patience and effort.

Kissing: Women love long passionate kisses. This foreplay move works the jaw muscles, tones the face, burns calories, and makes every nerve ending in the body tingle. An electrifying kiss can often feel hotter than sex, especially if you focus your mind on the scene. Create desire in your partner by supplying her with ample kisses on her mouth, and then stimulate multiple erogenous zones. Make her feel special and wanted. Additionally, why don't you continue to kiss her until she orgasms without touch?

SUMMARY

I hope that this guide has furnished you with many ideas on how to change your sex life from boring and tedious to simmering intense. Use the techniques in this guide and the power of your mind to focus on your needs, release tension, and allow your sexuality to take centre stage.

Take advantage of the many wonderful erogenous zones and the hottest one of all—the sexual mind. Alternatively, perhaps spend time with your partner and write a short horny story of your own.

I have described the methods on how to take charge of your sex life through spontaneity, building desire, flirting with your partner, and engaging in role-play to build excitement. I focused very much on foreplay and described its importance in building a long and fulfilling relationship.

The benefits of masturbation are clear in how regularly it allows you to become an effective lover by releasing your desire and multi-orgasmic potential. In the oral sex chapter, I gave fellatio and cunnilingus tips, and suggested having fun with sex toys in the bedroom.

I have also highlighted non-sexual techniques, primarily to help you appreciate foreplay and the fiery heat it creates in your senses. I will be very surprised if none of these techniques unleash your sexuality.

Try to stick to the "rules." They are detailed not only to help you to become an unselfish lover, but also to help you enjoy pleasure without the worry of giving anything but fervent moans in return. A good lover cares for his/her partner's sexual needs.

Conversation and desire is important and must be preserved in a long-term relationship or marriage. If you have no idea about your partner's needs, how will you be able to satisfy him/her sexually? Desire is important, and each of the seduction techniques can help to build this.

Couples who experiment with only missionary position will find a variety of fun positions in the "Sexual Workouts" chapter. If you want to tone the buttock and thigh muscles, there are many positions to offer that exact workout.

The aim of this fun guide is to teach you how to create intimacy with your partner and experience intensifying orgasms. The sexual mind is all about taking you and your partner to heightened states of ecstasy through the power of your mind— gaining knowledge of the hottest erogenous zones, writing hot erotica, watching your own homemade porn movies, dominating your partner, rubbing naked or fully clothed, massaging the scalp, and so much more. Use every tip, skill, and technique throughout this guide to become a better lover.

REFERENCES

[1] A sex session, often without foreplay, that lasts for less than five minutes.

[2] This act is oral sex of the penis.

[3] Stefan Bechtel, "Penis – Anatomy 101," in *The Practical Encyclopedia of Sex and Health,* ed. Alice Feinstein (New York City: St Martin's Press, 1993), pp. 236-237.

[4] Wikipedia, "Perineum," http://en.wikipedia.org/wiki/Perineum, accessed 4 September 2009.

[5] The tongue is used to stimulate the anus.

[6] This sexual act is also known as the rear entry position, where both anal and/or vaginal penetration can occur.

[7] Stefan Bechtel, "G-Spot," in *The Practical Encyclopedia of Sex and Health,* ed. Alice Feinstein (New York City: St Martin's Press, 1993), p. 140.

[8] Stefan Bechtel, "G-Spot – Female Ejaculation," in *The Practical Encyclopedia of Sex and Health,* ed. Alice Feinstein (New York City: St Martin's Press, 1993), p. 141.

[9] Positive Thinking Toolbox, "The Universal Law of Attraction and how it works with the other Universal Laws," http://www.positivethinking-toolbox.com/universal-law-of-attraction.html, accessed 13 March 2011.

[10] Smart Publications, "Pheromones: The Science Behind the Scent of Attraction," http://www.smart-publications.com/articles/view/human-pheromones-the-science-behind-the-scent-of-attraction/, accessed 6 September 2009.

[11] Holistic Health Articles, "Human Pheromone A Powerful Sexual Attractant,' http://www.holistichealtharticles.com/Artz/12965/336/Human-Pheromone-A-Powerful-Sexual-Attractant.html, accessed 21 January 2011.

[12] Smart Publications, "The Pheromone Revolution," http://www.smart-publications.com/articles/view/the-pheromone-revolution-sexual-attractants-and-their-effects-on-sex/, accessed 6 September 2009.

[13] Stefan Bechtel, "Sexual Smells – Search for the Pheromone," in *The Practical Encyclopedia of Sex and Health,* ed. Alice Feinstein (New York City: St Martin's Press, 1993), p. 295.

[14] Making other people laugh through insecurity or loneliness.

[15] Natural Skincare Authority, "Cosmetic Chemical Watch-List: The "A" to "Z" of Toxins in Skin Care," http://www.natural-skincare-authority.com/cosmetic-chemicals.html, accessed 13 March 2011.

[16] Organic Facts, "Health Benefits of Lemon Essential Oil," http://www.organicfacts.net/organic-oils/natural-essential-oils/health-benefits-of-lemon-oil.html, accessed 22 January 2011.

[17] Organic Facts, "Health Benefits of Vanilla Essential Oil," http://www.organicfacts.net/health-benefits/essential-oils/health-benefits-of-vanilla-essential-oil.html, accessed 22 January 2011.

[18] Tools for Wellness, "The Four Brain States," http://www.toolsforwellness.com/brainstates.html, accessed 25 January 2011.

[19] Stefan Bechtel, "Fantasy," in *The Practical Encyclopedia of Sex and Health*, ed. Alice Feinstein (New York City: St Martin's Press, 1993), p. 121.

[20] Wet and messy fetish that can include water and/or food play.

[21] This act is sexual intercourse with an animal.

[22] Stefan Bechtel, "Fantasy – Far Out Fantasy," in *The Practical Encyclopedia of Sex and Health*, ed. Alice Feinstein (New York City: St Martin's Press, 1993), p. 123.

[23] Sexual encounters that take place in a car park, where couples and single individuals can take part, or watch others make love in a very open environment.

[24] Wikipedia, "Cottaging," http://en.wikipedia.org/wiki/Cottaging, accessed 20 September 2010.

[25] Stefan Bechtel, "Orgasm – The Sexual Response Cycle," in *The Practical Encyclopedia of Sex and Health*, ed. Alice Feinstein (New York City: St Martin's Press, 1993), pp. 222-223.

[26] Stefan Bechtel, "Orgasm – Mysteries of the Female Orgasm," in *The Practical Encyclopedia of Sex and Health*, ed. Alice Feinstein (New York City: St Martin's Press, 1993), p. 224.

[27] White Lotus East, "Multiple Orgasm," http://www.whitelotuseast.com/MultipleOrgasm.htm, accessed 8 August 2010.

[28] Stefan Bechtel, "Orgasm – Multiple Orgasms: Can Men Learn How?" in *The Practical Encyclopedia of Sex and Health*, ed. Alice Feinstein (New York City: St Martin's Press, 1993), p. 226.

[29] Stefan Bechtel, "Desire – Low Sexual Desire," in *The Practical Encyclopedia of Sex and Health*, ed. Alice Feinstein (New York City: St Martin's Press, 1993), pp. 78-79.

[30] Stefan Bechtel, "Desire – Dissecting Desire," in *The Practical Encyclopedia of Sex and Health*, ed. Alice Feinstein (New York City: St Martin's Press, 1993), pp. 79-80.

[31] Stefan Bechtel, "Kissing – Scandalous Smooches," in *The Practical Encyclopedia of Sex and Health*, ed. Alice Feinstein (New York City: St Martin's Press, 1993), p. 183.

[32] Livestrong, "Kissing," http://www.livestrong.com/article/12470-kissing-/, accessed 17 September 2009.

[33] Wikipedia, "Body Language," http://en.wikipedia.org/wiki/Body_language, accessed 7 October 2010.

[34] Medicine Net, "Definition of Jugular vein," http://www.medterms.com/script/main/art.asp?articlekey=9187 accessed 2 November 2010.

[35] ExRx, "Quadratus Lumborum," http://www.exrx.net/Muscles/QuadratusLumborum.html accessed 2 November 2010.

[36] Right Health, "External Urethral Orifice (male)," http://www.righthealth.com/topic/External_urethral_orifice_(male), accessed 2 November 2010.

[37] Right Health, "Xiphoid Process," http://www.righthealth.com/topic/xiphoid_process, accessed 2 November 2010.

[38] Ivy Rose Holistic, "Zonula Ciliaris," http://www.ivy-rose.co.uk/References/glossary_entry446.htm, accessed 2 November 2010.

[39] This act is oral sex of the vagina.

[40] A couple who rub their feet together under a table to indicate sexual attraction or arousal.

[41] Stefan Bechtel, "Foreplay – Mistakes We Make," in *The Practical Encyclopedia of Sex and Health,* ed. Alice Feinstein (New York City: St Martin's Press, 1993), p. 131.

[42] Orgasmatron, "The Original Orgasmatron The Ultimate Head Massager!" http://www.orgasmatron.com.au/, accessed 3 November 2010.

[43] Schuelers, "Jungian Models of the Psyche," http://www.schuelers.com/ChaosPsyche/part_1_17.htm, accessed 15 August 2010.

[44] Boring sex sessions that require experimentation.

[45] IMDb, "Secretary," http://www.imdb.com/title/tt0274812/, accessed 17 September 2009.

[46] Heaven and Earth Home Remedies, "Urine Therapy, the p`energy of life and longevity!" http://www.heaven-and-earth-home-remedies.com/urine-therapy.html, accessed 21 March 2010.

[47] Articles Factory, "Urea –What Skin Care Benefits Does It Have?" http://www.articlesfactory.com/articles/health/urea-what-skin-care-benefits-does-it-have.html, accessed 17 August 2010.

[48] Stefan Bechtel, "Masturbation," in *The Practical Encyclopedia of Sex and Health,* ed. Alice Feinstein (New York City: St Martin's Press, 1993), p. 197.

[49] EFT Universe, "EFT: Healing the Emotional Roots of Disease," http://www.eftuniverse.com/, accessed 23 March 2010.

[50] 4 Men, "Over Masturbation," http://www.4-men.org/overmasturbation.html, accessed 5 February 2011.

[51] Herbal Love, "Effects of Over Masturbation In Women," http://www.herballove.com/article.asp?art=552, accessed 5 February 2011.

[52] Stefan Bechtel, "Masturbation – What is "Excessive," in *The Practical Encyclopedia of Sex and Health*, ed. Alice Feinstein (New York City: St Martin's Press, 1993), pp. 199-200.

[53] Oral sex with another person, performed at opposite ends to pleasure both the male and female genitals.

[54] Psychic 101, "Telepathic Influence and Remote Hypnosis," http://www.psychic101.com/telepathy-influence.html, accessed 7 February 2011.

[55] Mystic Mouse, "Who Is The Higher Self?" http://www.mystic-mouse.co.uk/Wisdom_Texts/Mystic_Visions/Higher_Self.htm, accessed 7 February 2011.

[56] New Brain New World, "Kundalini and Sex," http://www.newbrainnewworld.com/?Awakening_of_Kundalini:Kundalini_and_S ex, accessed 30 August 2010.

Proof

Made in the USA
Charleston, SC
12 April 2011